BUDGET FRIENDLY COLLEGE COOKBOOK

+125 Super easy and healthy recipes for every student ready in 15 minutes with 5 $ or less.

EMILY ANDERSON

TABLE OF CONTENTS

Introduction

Food.

It's something we all think about every day, even multiple times a day. It's a necessity. It's a delicacy. It's energy and fuel. It's a treat. It's the center of celebrations, the heart of family and friend gatherings.

It can also be a hassle for some people. Expensive, time-consuming, and difficult to prepare.

But it doesn't have to be that way. Good food—healthy, delicious, tasty, nutritious, satisfying—can also be simple food.

And simple is key in college. Most college students juggle very busy schedules, including classes, homework, jobs, friends, family, sports, clubs, or other extra-curricular activities. Adding cooking and eating into that mix can be stressful.

The purpose of this cookbook is to relieve the USU student's stress in at least one area— food. This cookbook is filled with recipes designed for busy college students who may not have a lot of time to cook or a lot of money to buy food.

It also has some great resources beyond just recipes. Included is a list of cooking terms and definitions, tips for grocery shopping, a helpful method for making your meals healthy and balanced, and other tips and tricks to make preparing and eating meals the least of your worries

CHAPTER
1

Did you know that households in the UK spend an average of £57 a week on food and drink? This number increases to £75 when you factor in dining out, as revealed in a recent report by the Office for National Statistics.

Instead of sacrificing the quality of food, we've listed 10 tips that will help save you money on your wining and dining.

10 Tips For Eating On A Tiny Budget

1.   Consider Where To Shop

If you don't live near a supermarket, you're probably making frequent trips to the local corner shop. Making one weekly trip to a supermarket will reduce your weekly food shop cost and increase the variety of your ingredients.

If you live in the city, consider heading to your local fruit and veg market as produce is often fresher and cheaper than supermarkets.

2.   When To Shop

Always check the reduced shelves. Meats with a day left on their' use by date' are perfect when eaten straight away or, if you prefer to buy in bulk, freezing for up to 3 months.

Never food shop when you're hungry; statistics show you will part with more of your hard-earned cash.

3.   Check The Price

Make sure you check the price 'per kg' and choose the cheaper option. This is particularly effective when comparing packaged or loose fruit and vegetables. As if saving money wasn't enough of a draw, loose is better for the planet as less packaging means less waste. Pre-trimmed vegetables or ready-grated cheese are certainly more expensive. Remember, it takes seconds to trim your vegetables, but it takes hours to earn a living.

4.   Buy Own-Brand

You can eat and drink premium without the price tag. Blind taste tests have shown that cheaper supermarket branded food often trumps household names. Often, the only difference between basic and premium is in the packaging and marketing budget. This doesn't just apply to food: supermarkets also do their version of wines and spirits.

5.   Buy In Bulk

If your weekly budget can stretch to it, buy bigger packs of long-life ingredients like rice, canned food, frozen produce, and toilet paper. This often reduces the per-portion price. If you live in shared accommodation, consider banding together to bulk-buy household items – it'll benefit you all.

6.   Buy In Season

This one is a bit of a no-brainer, but when fruit and vegetables hit peak production, their price is often slashed. Consider when and what you're shopping for to make every penny work as hard as it can.

7.   Cook Once, Eat Twice

Cooking extra for the next day (or to freeze for later) will save you money and time. Taking a packed lunch to work can save as much as £1000 each year!

8.   Buy Big Flavors

Identify the flavors you like and add them to your meals regularly. This way, expensive meat doesn't have to be at the center of a meal; less is more. Some cheap ingredients that are big on flavor include eggs, stock, olive oil, sesame oil, bacon, tinned sardines, soy sauce, lemon, lime, chili flakes, coconut milk, garam masala, Chinese five-spice, coriander, and ginger.

9.   Make Meat Go Further

Before you buy the popular cuts, remember that there are equally (if not more) delicious cuts that are cheaper. Chicken thighs are more succulent than breast, can contain bones, which is great for homemade stock and soups, and can have beautiful skin that you can grill until crisp.

Beef shin and brisket are brilliant when slow-cooked in soups and stews, and consider picking up cooking bacon (500g for 60p, Tesco) – these are part rashers of all shapes and sizes.

10.   Freeze, Freeze, Freeze

We've already mentioned making extra and freezing your meals for another day, but here are some additional tips to make you love your freezer:

- Buy plastic takeaway containers with lids and freezer proof sandwich bags with ties.
- Label your frozen produce: it'll help you keep on top of everything!
- Cool cooked food before freezing and aim to get food into the freezer within two hours of cooking.
- As a general rule, freeze items for up to three months and use the oldest items first.
- Defrost food in the fridge by taking it out the night before. As a general rule, be sure to use defrosted food within 24 hours.
- Always ensure frozen food is piping hot before eating, and once defrosted, never re-freeze.

CHAPTER 2
Kitchen Skills Are The Key To Great Food

Everyone, young or old, can enjoy having a handy collection of basic cooking skills with a little practice. Mastering this list can help you make better meals, save time, be safer in the kitchen, and just plain have fun!

- Do Pasta Right

The difference between rookie- and restaurant-quality pasta is just a little pasta water, salt, finesse, and maybe butter (OK, often butter.) Your pasta-cooking water should taste like the ocean: salty. This seemingly obscene quantity of salt is crucial, as it will flavor your noodles. Cook your pasta al dente (meaning it still has some bite to it). Before you dump it out, save some water: it's loaded with all the beautiful starches from your pasta that will naturally make any sauce you add it to creamier. Finish off your pasta in a sauté pan with whatever sauce you desire, plus some of that pasta water. This way, the sauce will be creamier and will better bind to your pasta. And adding a little butter at the end never made anything worse. Once you've got the basics down, try these ridiculously easy weeknight pasta dinners!

- Know Three Ways To Cook Eggs

Eating fried eggs every morning can get boring fast. But once you can scramble (recipe here!), poach, soft boil, hard boil (recipe here!), or make an omelet (recipe here!) or frittata, no day will be the same. You probably know how to scramble or fry an egg, so we recommend mastering poached eggs and the omelet.
They are the two most sophisticated eggs form,s and you'll be sure to impress any date or friend if they're lucky enough to find themselves at your place for Breakfast-Breakfast or brunch.

- Make Pan Sauce

Pan sauces are quick and easy to take your roasted chicken or pasta to the next level. If you've roasted or seared a piece of meat, the little brown bits at the bottom are solid gold. Hit them with a little wine, garlic, and chicken stock, and within minutes you'll have a ridiculously delicious sauce.
 Other quick sauces can consist of tomatoes, basil, olives; white wine, shallots, and tarragon; or the classic lemon, capers, and brown butter. Add a dab of cold butter at the end, off the heat, to emulsify your sauce and make it extra delicious.

- Make A Vinaigrette

Store-bought salad dressings are for punks and stars of Cool Hand Luke. They are loaded with sugars and so many unnecessary ingredients that allow them to sit on the shelf for ages. Instead, make your own. Vinaigrettes have two basic components: acid and fat. Acid is usually vinegar or citrus, and the fat is often a type of vegetable oil. They work on a 1:3 ratio of vinegar to oil or 1:2 for milder acids such as lemon juice. Throw in some salt and Pepper, and you have a basic vinaigrette. Add mustard to help bind the mixture and add some flavor. Then get creative. Mix up the vinegar and oils, add honey, shallots, ginger, soy sauce, and herbs. Consider Newman owned.

- Sharpen Knives

Fun fact: dull knives are more dangerous than sharp ones and are more likely to slip when cutting because they don't have a defined edge. So don't keep dull knives. There are three main ways to handle sharpening: use a sharpening stone, use a manual or electric sharpener, or send your knives out. The pros all use stones, but it requires some technique and time.

A sharpener is easy enough to use, but if you are super lazy, just send them out. Warning: professional sharpeners tend to take a lot off the knife, so your knife's lifespan may decrease. Not sure if your knives are dull? Carefully run the blade over your thumbnail. If it catches, you have a sharp knife. If it glides right over, it's dull as hell. Now go and sharpen it.

- Handle a knife

Basic knife skills are an integral part of cooking. Yes, you may say you can avoid any knife work by buying pre-made sauces, soups, or the like, but then you ain't cooking, and it's not fresh, and you're no better than an 18-year-old college boy. Learn how to hold a knife properly so you don't cut off your fingers and start slicing and dicing. Cutting up onion is a great place to start. Congratulations, you are now an adult.

- Make A Chicken Cutlet.

The chicken cutlet is like chicken fingers for grown-ups. And who doesn't love chicken fingers? The proper breading technique requires four steps: 1) season your chicken; 2) dip it in flour; 3) dip it in eggs; 4) dip it in breadcrumbs. Then fry or bake it. If using a chicken breast, we recommend pounding it or slicing it in half to ensure a crispy-yet-moist cutlet. We prefer skinless, boneless chicken thighs, but that's your call.

Once you've mastered this basic principle, countless variations are at your disposal. You can substitute chicken with almost any protein, from pork and beef (think chicken-fried steak) to fish and even tofu, and serve it over rice or salads, in wraps, sandwiches, and more. With a few simple variations and help from your foreign-language buddy, you can be cooking up Milanese, schnitzel, or katsu (here's a Cap'n Crunch Chicken Katsu recipe for the bold). Sounds fancier than just a cutlet, right?

- Properly Wash Vegetables

Unless you exclusively buy triple-washed baby kale, chances are your vegetables and lettuce are dirty. No one wants to bite into grit or sand, so clean them well. Fill two big bowls with cold water, and then let your veggie of choice take a dip. Swoosh it around well, then lift it. All the dirt will sink to the bottom. Transfer your greens to the other bowl. Dump out the dirty water and refill with fresh water. Repeat this process until your water is crystal clear. For quick and efficient drying, indulge in a salad spinner. Voila.

- Make Some Baked Goods.

You're almost 30, and let's face it: those PTA meetings and bake sales are right around the corner. Don't be that parent who brings in cardboard donuts from the gas station. Instead, a master at least one baked good and make it you're go-to. Cookies are great because you can keep all of the ingredients in your pantry and refrigerator for a long time. Banana bread, pumpkin bread, and brownies (try this recipe) are other easy crowd-pleasers. Bonus: baking makes your home smell amazing.

- Roast Vegetables

When vegetables surpass 280 degrees, something beautiful happens. Thanks to Maillard reactions and naturally occurring sugars and amino acids, the vegetables start to brown and develop a beautiful, more intense flavor. And the best part? To roast vegetables, all you have to do is preheat your oven to around 425 degrees, chop up your vegetable of choice, toss it with some oil and salt, and pop it in! We recommend using parchment paper or a silicone mat on your baking sheet for easier clean-up. And remember, water boils at 212. Therefore wet vegetables can never brown, so keep those veggies nice and dry!

- Season Food

In the culinary world, "season" means salt. Properly seasoning your food is crucial to locking in flavor and making your food tasty. It's important to salt your food throughout the cooking process, not just at the end. Big pieces of meat such as thick steaks and roasts require a ton of salt to help develop that golden crust we so love. But be careful: you can always add more salt at the end, but you can never un-salt your food.

- Sauté Stuff

The art of the sauté is quick, insanely flavorful, and fun. To do it successfully, put your pan on the burner, turn up the flame as hot as hell, add your oil, allow it to heat up, and don't crowd your pan with too many veggies. Ignore any of these tips, and you'll never attain that golden sear you so desire.

- Shock And Blanch Vegetables

Vegetable cuisine is vast, filled with so many possibilities: shocking and blanching your greens opens you up to so many of them. The concept is simple. Bring a pot of salted water to a roaring boil. Add your vegetables, making sure they are more or less of the same size and type to ensure even cooking. Cook until they're tender with a little bite (adjusting to your preference), and then, using a strainer or tongs, immediately place them in a big bath of ice water.

This polar bear plunge abruptly stops the cooking process and locks their color and texture in place. From here, you can enjoy a lovely vegetable salad or go on to dry and then sauté your vegetables, making them crispy yet tender. This technique works great for herbs if you are making purees and want them to be green.

- Thicken Sauces

Nobody likes a runny sauce. The general desired consistency for a sauce is "napping," meaning "coating": you want your sauce to coat your food and your mouth. There are many ways to thicken up a sauce, but our favorite three techniques are: 1) reduce; 2) use a cornstarch slurry; 3) add beurre manié.

Reduce: Reducing your sauce works best when one of its main components is animal stock (i.e., chicken or veal). Over time the natural gelatin in the stock will cause it to thicken and become glorious. Veal stock is higher in gelatin than chicken and makes for the richest sauces. Reduce your sauce slowly, over a gentle simmer, and be sure to skim it for any impurities on the surface. Be careful not to over-reduce, or it may become too salty or too thick, almost like glue.

Cornstarch Slurry: A slurry is a fun word for a semi-liquid mixture and is a classic American go-to for thickening sauces. To make a slurry:

- Combine Regular Cornstarch And Cold Water.
- Add equal parts water to the corn starch, mixing it well with a fork or small whisk to ensure no lumps.
- Slowly drizzle your slurry into your sauce while whisking it over heat until it bubbles,

thus activating the thickening agents.

Usually, you want about one tablespoon of slurry mixture per cup of liquid you want to thicken. Be sure to adjust your seasoning as you've slightly diluted your sauce. And yes, this method is gluten-free.

Beurre Manié: Beurre manié is like a roux but made with your hands (it translates to kneaded butter). Work very room-temperature butter with equal parts flour until you make a paste. Drop this concoction into your sauce and whisk very well, letting it come up to a boil, activating the thickening agents while cooking out the flour flavor. Now you have a thickened and buttery sauce. And, once again, butter is a good thing.

- Make Chocolate Sauce

Strawberries dipped in a rich chocolate sauce is the classic sexiest dessert, and it happens to be the easiest one. It would help if you had chocolate pieces or chips, heavy cream, and a double boiler to make your chocolate sauce. Create a double boiler, take a small saucepan, add some water to it, and cover it with a metal or glass bowl (plastic will melt, obviously). You want there to be some space between the bowl and the water. Bring the water up to a light simmer. Add the chocolate and heavy cream and stir until melted. And that's it.

- Cook Three Basic Meals

In the process of learning the previous skills, you've probably picked up a dish or two to work on. Master three basic meals, and you'll be set for dinner parties, potlucks, and general entertaining while still keeping it exciting for yourself. Once you've truly become comfortable with the techniques necessary to execute the dishes, you can start to experiment and get creative. Now you're cooking.

- Keep Your Kitchen Safe And Clean.

Accomplishing everything above is great but worthless if you can't keep your kitchen clean. The best way to maintain a healthy and manageable kitchen is to clean up as you go. Always wipe down surfaces and appliances after use. There are all sorts of antibacterial soaps and bleaches at your disposal to spray as you go.

Distilled vinegar is a wonderful natural disinfectant and is incredibly versatile for all your cleaning needs. When handling raw meats and fish, try to wear gloves and make sure to wash and disinfect your cutting boards and knives thoroughly. Don't forget to regularly clean out the refrigerator and wipe it down as well. Lord knows it's time to throw out that half-eaten yogurt from two months ago.

- Don't Shop When You're Hungry

If you go to the grocery store hungry, you are more likely to stray from your grocery list and buy something on impulse.

When you're hungry, you often crave foods that aren't good for you or your budget. Try to grab a piece of fruit, yogurt, or another healthy snack before you go to the store.

- Buy Whole Foods

Some foods are way cheaper in a less processed form. For example, a block of cheese is cheaper than shredded cheese, and canned beans are cheaper than refried ones.

Whole grains, like brown rice and oats, are also cheaper per serving than most processed cereals. The less processed foods are also often sold in larger quantities and yield more servings per package.

- Buy Generic Brands

Most stores offer generic brands for nearly any product. All food manufacturers have to follow standards to provide safe food. The generic brands may be the same quality as other national brands, just less expensive.

However, read the ingredients lists to make sure that you're not getting a product of lower quality than you're used to.

8. Stop Buying Junk Food

Cut out some of the junk food from your diet. You would be surprised to see how much you may be paying for soda, crackers, cookies, prepackaged meals, and processed foods.

Even though they offer very little nutrition and are packed with unhealthy ingredients, they are also very expensive. By skipping the processed and unhealthy foods, you can spend more of your budget on higher-quality, healthy foods.

- Stock Up On Sales

If you have favorite products or staples that you use frequently, you should stock up on them when they're on sale.

If you're sure that it's something you'll use, you may as well stock up and save a little money.

Just make sure that it will last for a while and won't expire in the meantime. It will not save you any money to buy something you'll end up throwing out later on.

- Buy Cheaper Cuts of Meat

Fresh meat and fish can be quite expensive.

However, you can get many cuts of meat that cost way less. These are great to use in burritos, casseroles, soups, stews, and stir-fries. It may also help buy a large and inexpensive cut of meat to use in several different meals during the week.

- Replace Meat With Other Proteins

Eating less meat may be a good way to save money. Try having one or two days per week to use other protein sources, such as legumes, hemp seeds, eggs, or canned fish. These are all very inexpensive, nutritious, and easy to prepare. Most of them also have a long shelf life and are therefore less likely to spoil quickly.

- Shop For Produce That Is In Season

Local produce that is in season is generally cheaper. It is also usually at its peak in both nutrients and flavor. Produce that is not in the season has often been transported halfway around the world to get to your store, which is not good for your environment or budget.

Also, buy produce by the bag if you can. That is usually a lot cheaper than buying by the piece. If you buy more than you need, you can freeze the rest or incorporate it into next week's meal plans.

- Buy Frozen Fruits And Vegetables

Fresh fruits, berries, and vegetables are usually in season only a few months per year and are sometimes rather expensive.

Quick-frozen produce is usually just as nutritious. It is cheaper, available all year, and is usually sold in large bags.Frozen produce is great to use when cooking, making smoothies, or as toppings for oatmeal or yogurt.

Furthermore, you gain the advantage of taking out only what you're about to use. The rest will be kept safe from spoiling in the freezer. Reducing produce waste is a great way to save money.

- Buy In Bulk

Buying some foods in bulk quantities can save you a lot of money. Grains, such as brown rice, millet, barley, and oats, are all available in bulk. They also keep for a long time if you store them in airtight containers.

This is also true for beans, lentils, some nuts, and dried fruit. These are all staple foods that are relatively inexpensive and can be used in various healthy meals.

- Grow Your Produce

If you can, it is a great idea to grow your produce. Seeds are very cheap to buy. With some time and effort, you may be able to grow your herbs, sprouts, tomatoes, onions, and many more delicious crops. Having a continuous supply at home saves you money at the store. Home-grown produce may also taste a lot better than the store-bought varieties. You can also guarantee that it is picked at the peak of ripeness.

- Pack Your Lunch

Eating out is very expensive, especially if done regularly. Packing your lunch, snacks, drinks and other meals are less expensive and way healthier than eating out.

If you have adapted to cooking large meals at home, you'll always have a steady lunch to bring with you without any additional effort or cost. It does require some planning, but it should save you a lot of money at the end of the month.

- Use Coupons Wisely

Coupons are a great way to save some money. Just be sure to use them wisely. Most coupons are for unhealthy, processed foods.

Sort out the good quality deals from the junk, stock up on cleaning products, healthy foods, and other staples you'll use.

By cutting the cost of products needed around the house, you can spend more of your budget on healthy foods.

- Appreciate Less Expensive Foods

There are a lot of foods available that are both inexpensive and healthy.

By making some adjustments and using ingredients that you may not be used to, you can prepare many delicious and inexpensive meals.

Try increasing your use of eggs, beans, seeds, frozen fruits and vegetables, cheaper cuts of meat, and whole grains. These all taste great, are cheap (especially in bulk), and very nutritious.

- Buy From Cheap, Online Retailers

Several online retailers offer healthy foods for up to 50% cheaper. By registering, you get access to daily discounts and deals.

What's more, the products are then delivered straight to your door. Thrive Market is a very good online retailer that focuses exclusively on healthy and unprocessed foods. Buying as much as you can from them can save you money.

CHAPTER 4
The Art Of Storage

When you think of storing food for later, what comes to mind? Do you imagine wrapping up some leftovers, putting them in the fridge, and calling it a day? If you're a more advanced practitioner of the art of food storage, you might fill your crisper drawer with veggies and keep a few fruits on the counter to ripen. But what else should you know about how to preserve and store food, and why does it even matter?

Why Proper Food Storage Matters
- Here are some of the benefits when you get good at storing food:
- You reduce food waste, which saves money and is better for the environment.
- Fruits and vegetables will stay fresh longer.
- You can buy things in bulk or in season, which will save money. And you can use them over a longer period without rushing, which can reduce stress.
- You can treat yourself to fruits and veggies at all times of the year.
- Old-time methods of food storage can make for a fun hobby! Or a creative new way to eat your fruits and veggies.
- You can eat well during a power outage or while camping, as many food storage techniques, don't require electricity.
- One traditional method of food preservation, fermenting, can add beneficial microbes to your diet.

Three Types Of Food
All food can be classified into one of three groups, which require different storage methods.
1. Perishable Foods
These include many raw fruits and vegetables and those who eat them, meat, dairy, and eggs. All cooked foods are considered perishable foods. To store these foods for any length of time, perishable foods need to be held at refrigerator or freezer temperatures. Many perishable foods should be used within 3-7 days (less for many animal products) if refrigerated.

2. Semi-Perishable Foods
Food that's semi-perishable — depending on how they're stored and handled — can go bad quickly or can have an extended shelf life. Flour, grain products, dried fruits, and dry mixes are considered semi-perishable. If optimally stored and handled, like in a clean, vacuum-sealed bag, semi-perishable foods may remain unspoiled for six months to a year. Frozen, some can last even longer.

3. Staple Or Non-Perishable Foods
Dried beans, spices, and canned goods are all non-perishable foods. They won't spoil unless they're handled carelessly. However, even if they're stored under ideal conditions, they can

start to lose quality over extended periods.

Factors That Affect Food Storage Life

For perishable and semi-perishable foods, the general rule of thumb is that it needs to be stored or preserved if you can't use it promptly.

Here are the main factors that will impact a food's shelf life during storage:

•   The food itself (for example, strawberries can degrade in as little as a day, while potatoes can last for months when properly stored).

•   The freshness and ripeness of the food when you obtain it. This depends in part on where it was grown and how long it spent in transit. Even if you just bought it from a grocery store, it may have been just very recently harvested… or not.

•   The length of time and the temperature at which it was held before you bought it. Whether it's the refrigerator, freezer, countertop, pantry, or basement, the temperature of your food storage areas.

•   The humidity level in your food storage areas (which can vary greatly depending on location in your house and what region you live in)

•   The type of storage container or packaging the food is stored in, such as glass, plastic, foil, or cloth.

The Pros And Cons Of 6 Ways To Store Food

There are numerous ways to store food, each with its benefits and downsides. Here are some things to consider, depending on which method you're using.

1.   Canning

Canning can be a cost-effective way to preserve the quality of food at home. Commonly canned foods include applesauce, vegetables, jams and jellies, and baby purees.

The basic steps for proper canning include thoroughly washing the fresh produce you'll be using, peeling and hot packing if needed, adding acids like lemon juice or vinegar if the food isn't already sufficiently acidic using self-sealing containers with lids. Canning jars are then processed by boiling water (for acidic fruits and vegetables) or using a pressure canner (for low-acid fruits and vegetables) for the appropriate amount of time. This helps prevent bacterial growth and kills any pathogens to ensure safety.

Home canning can lead to significant financial savings, and it gives you no risk of BPA contamination, as you will use glass mason jars in place of plastic or BPA-lined commercial cans.

Canned foods also keep their nutritional value longer, though some losses do occur. Approximately 30-50% of vitamins A, C, thiamin, and riboflavin are lost during the healing process, with an additional 5-20% loss of these per year. Less sensitive vitamins remain intact over time and are found in only slightly lower amounts than in fresh food. Vegetables can be pretty hardy if handled and canned quickly and can maintain much of their nutrition. And you don't necessarily need to do anything with canned foods before eating — you can just enjoy them right out of the container.

- Risks & Downsides Of Canning

There are also some risks to consider with canning. Home canning requires a sterile environment to prevent contamination. Canned foods also need to be stored at the right temperatures — with airtight lids — to prevent pathogens like botulism. In other words, don't rely solely on the instructions in this article. Follow these USDA guidelines and pay attention to cleanliness, timing, and temperature to ensure you're preserving food and not armies of harmful microbes.

There are a couple of potential downsides to canning as well. Aside from losing some of their flavor and nutrients over the years, canned preserves, jams, and jellies often use a lot of added sugar in their preservation process, presenting some health concerns.

It's important to be aware that mold can grow on canned foods, especially on the surfaces of high sugar foods like jams and jellies. Mold can produce toxic compounds called mycotoxins, which may be carcinogenic. Luckily, mold is often colorful and easy to see on canned food surfaces. You can prevent mold through proper heat processing and airtight sealing practices. It's a good idea to test your canning jars' seals before putting them away for storage in the cupboard or garage.

2. Freezing

A great option for preserving most foods. You can freeze soups, baby purees, oats, and coffee grounds to veggie burger patties, chopped fruit, and blanched vegetables.

A properly maintained freezer will store food for long periods, after which you can safely thaw (either in the fridge or by setting it in cold water only) and cook it as desired. Nutritionally, foods that you prepare at home and then freeze are almost always better for you than frozen meals you'd find at the grocery store.

Freezing comes with minimal risks, but there are a few things to keep in mind. Everything in the freezer is subject to freezer burn, which happens when air comes in contact with the food's surface, and it can look like grayish-brown spots. This doesn't make the food unsafe to eat, but it does make it dry in certain areas. You can cut these areas off when you thaw the food. And while some foods taste very similar after freezing, others go through significant and sometimes not altogether pleasant texture changes.

And as much as we'd like them to, frozen foods don't have an infinite shelf life. Foods such as soups and stews, vegetables, and fruits can spoil after a long enough time. To prevent storing foods in the back of your freezer and forgetting about them for three generations ("Hey, isn't this a piece of grandma and grandpa's wedding cake?") and risking spoilage (which I'm guilty of!), write the date on the container in permanent marker and use or toss extremely old specimens regularly. I'd recommend storing more recently frozen foods at the back and choosing to thaw and eat the older items first. This creates a natural rotation and cuts down on eventual food waste.

3.   Drying or Dehydration

An excellent preservation method for fruits, vegetables, and herbs. Drying food tends to increase its flavor, costs very little, and makes storage easier by reducing its size.

How does it work? Dehydration removes water from fresh food, which prevents bacterial growth. The moisture content of home-dried food should be around 20% or less. You can do this by using a commercial dehydrator, hanging bunches of fresh herbs to dry (unless you live in a high humidity area), oven drying foods, or even using the sun to make your solar food dryer. Before you dry certain fruits and vegetables, you may want to blanch them (dip them briefly in boiling water) to help preserve them.

However, dehydration does have some drawbacks. While many nutrients remain fairly stable during dehydration, vitamins A, C, and thiamin are sensitive to heat (if the produce is blanched or heated in the oven) and air.

Also, electric dehydrators use a lot of energy, which you can avoid using some of the other home drying methods when possible. Dehydrating food can also take a while — often over ten hours — so be sure you're prepared to be patient and do some planning ahead if you pursue this method. And preparing foods for drying can take time, too. For example, slicing and coring fruits and spreading them out on a drying rack, all of which may need to be done manually.

4.   Fermentation

Fermenting foods is a great way to boost your intake of healthy probiotics (good bacteria) that are great for your digestive system and immunity. Fermenting starts with Lacto-fermentation, which is a bacterial process that preserves and boosts nutrients in food. The basic steps include chopping, grating, or otherwise preparing your raw food, deciding on the culture you'll use (typically salt, whey, or starter culture), preparing and adding brine, and placing everything in an airtight container in a cold environment.

Fermentation does require some care, as food can go bad during this process if you're not using fresh veggies or don't use distilled or purified water. Fermenting also typically uses salt, as salt helps preserve food by drawing out its water content and preventing bacterial formation. This is a drawback for people. You may want to think of fresh sauerkraut, kimchi, and other salty fermented vegetables as the "salt source" for some meals.

5.   A Note About Mold

How do you tell if fermented foods have gone bad? Often, a film may develop on the surface, but this may not necessarily be mold. Sometimes it's a harmless yeast called kahm yeast. Sometimes, fuzzy spots on your pink, black, green, or red food are mold. This doesn't mean the whole batch is garbage, though, as you can often remove the top layer and still safely consume what's underneath the brine — if it smells and tastes OK. However, I always say, "When in doubt, throw it out." (Or better yet, put it in the compost!)

Mold is fairly rare in fermented foods, and there are some ways to prevent it from developing. First, use the freshest produce you can; an ideal world would be organic from your garden. Next, choose the appropriate cool temperature for fermentation, between 65-70 degrees Fahrenheit. Using the right amount of salt — around 1-3 tablespoons per quart of water — can help prevent mold.

6.   Pickling

Similar to fermentation, pickling can be done on more than just cucumbers. Have you ever had pickled green beans? Yum! Some other commonly pickled foods include beets, cauliflower, peppers, cabbage, and even fruits like lemon or mango.

Pickling preserves food in a high-acid solution, either via a process of natural fermentation or by adding vinegar and salt (and sometimes sugar). It prevents spoilage and extends shelf life. Many combinations of pickled foods also look pretty and make great gifts!

Very few ingredients are needed for home pickling. All you need are:

The fruit or vegetable.

- A high-acid brine solution (water, vinegar, salt, and optional sugar).
- An airtight container.

6.	Cold Storage

This is the most common way many of us store produce, whether in the refrigerator or an underground root cellar if you're lucky enough to have one of those. Cold storage products, like apples, pears, root vegetables, celery, and cabbage, can last several months if stored correctly.

It's important to make sure you're aware of and following ideal temperatures and conditions for food storage to get the best shelf life from them. For example, Apples should ideally be stored at just above freezing in a damp and breathable bag.

Even though it's tempting to bring your fresh produce home and line it all up on the counter, it's best not to store things closely together as this can cause them to spoil. Many fruits and vegetables, like apples, cantaloupe, blueberries, bananas, potatoes, and tomatoes, give off ethylene gas, making things around them ripen and brown faster.

Different fruits and veggies need to be stored in particular ways to preserve their freshness best. Some produce like apricots, grapes, strawberries, green onions, and asparagus go in the fridge right away. Avocados, kiwi, peaches, and pears should ripen on the counter before you put them in the fridge. And never refrigerate pomegranates, mandarin oranges, ginger, and jicama, as they are best at room temperature.

7.	Other Things To Keep In Mind With Cold Storage

Maintaining the proper amount of moisture is also important to prevent drying out, wilting, or premature mold. Rather than storing produce right on the counter or shelf, it helps store them in containers with holes to promote air circulation like baskets, mesh, or paper bags with holes punched in them.

If your fridge has a fan, as most do, it can dry foods out. The produce drawer is typically protected from this effect. Foods stored loose in the fridge, outside of the produce drawer will dry out if not kept in a bag, container, or otherwise protected from the fan's drying effect.

Choosing good-looking produce at the store also helps prevent early spoilage. If you're not going to eat them immediately, don't buy avocados that are already mushy or bananas that are already spotting. Check your produce to make sure it's not badly bruised, discolored, punctured, or otherwise damaged.

It's also important to wait to wash produce until you're ready to preserve, cook, or eat it,

CHAPTER 5
Kitchen Equipment

If you've ever attempted to purchase cookware for a new kitchen or tried to improve the quality of tools in your current kitchen, you've probably found that stocking up on high-\ quality kitchen essentials is much more difficult than it should be.

And this makes sense, doesn't it? Nowadays, everywhere we look, someone tells us to buy their product that will supposedly make our lives easier. I'm sure all of the following sound familiar:

- Cooking TV show hosts recommending their products
- Branded cooking sets from your favorite celebrity chef
- Kitchen stores stocking unusual, "one-trick-pony" items
- Infomercials are aggressively selling cheap gizmos.
- Kitchen websites are promoting every item as a "must-have."

And so on. Instead of all this increased choice making our lives easier, it's made it that much more difficult to separate the quality from the junk. We decided to test all the kitchen equipment we could get our hands on to solve this problem and make stocking a minimalist, high-quality kitchen as easy as possible.

- The Best Minimalist Kitchen Essentials

When we started our cooking journey, we were full of confusion and frustration as we began our search for the best cookware and essential kitchen tools for minimalist cooks. When you start with no knowledge, the learning curve is immense.

But after years of refining our cooking techniques, creating and testing simple recipes, learning how to plan our meals, and building a customizable meal planning service for busy folks like us, we learned exactly which tools one needs (and doesn't need) to stock a fully functional and multi-purpose minimalist kitchen.

Note: We've tried to make it easy to navigate this kitchen essentials list and find what you need right away.

That is, except those rare items that combine such high-quality and great value that they stand alone as a clear winner.

Let's dig into the best high quality and versatile kitchen essentials that provide the most value for your money.

- The Best Minimalist Kitchen Essentials:

Cookware, Utensils, Equipment, Tools, Appliances & More

When we started our cooking journey, we were full of confusion and frustration as we began our search for the best cookware and essential kitchen tools for minimalist cooks. When you start with no knowledge, the learning curve is immense.

But after years of refining our cooking techniques, creating and testing simple recipes, learning how to plan our meals, and building a customizable meal planning service for busy folks like us, we learned exactly which tools one needs (and doesn't need) to stock a fully functional and multi-purpose minimalist kitchen.

And each of these categories contains items that are categorized into recommended, premium, and budget picks. That is, except those rare items that combine such high-quality and great value that they stand alone as a clear winner.

Let's dig into the best high quality and versatile kitchen essentials that provide the most value for your money.

- Chef's Knife

If you've only ever used a cheap chef's knife for your cooking needs, switching to a high-quality knife will be a night and day difference. Seriously, when we upgraded to a high-quality chef's knife, we couldn't believe how much sharper, heavier, and easier it was to cut and chop with the quality knife. And since you can use a chef's knife for all of your cutting needs (and use it every time you cook), one high-quality purchase will serve you for years to come.

- Cutting Board

One of the most basic tools you need in your kitchen is a good cutting board. You'll be using it every time you cook (just like your chef's knife), so it's important to choose one that's durable and well designed.

The good grips cutting board is dishwasher safe and is built from odor-resistant polypropylene - meaning it will last a long time. Pick this inexpensive cutting board up, and you won't regret it.

- Cutting Board (Premium)

Now, if you're looking for the Ferrari of cutting boards, look no further than this Proteak edge grain cutting board. If you haven't tried a cutting board like this before, it'll be hard to understand just how different - and how much higher quality - it is. But we can confirm that upgrading to a cutting board like this will bring you joy in the kitchen every time you use it.

You have to take better care of this cutting board than our plastic recommendation; by cleaning it immediately after use and avoiding the dishwasher. But this item is unique and will last you a long time, so if you're ready for an upgrade from the usual plastic cutting boards most home cooks sport nowadays, this one gets our vote.

- Can Opener

It's not often that a piece of cookware brings you joy every time you use it. But that's exactly what this can opener from Kuhn Rikon does! This 5-in-1 can opener pulls tabs, crowns caps, unscrews tops, and opens jar lids and cans safely,

- Measuring Cups

Measuring cups are used for precisely measuring the volume of liquid or solid cooking ingredients. You may not think that measuring cups can be anything special. Any set will do, right? Well, as it turns out, great design can extend down to measuring cups. This stackable set of measuring cups from Kitchenmade has all sorts of smart features that eliminate the small frustrations that measuring cups often bring about.

- Measuring Spoons

Measuring spoons are used to precisely measure smaller amounts of liquid or solid cooking ingredients than measuring cups. This set of 5 stainless steel measuring spoons from Prepworks contains measurements of ¼ tsp up to 1 tbsp. They're magnetic and nested, so you can easily put them away without losing any of them (which can often happen for the smaller spoons).

They're also designed to be double-sided to accommodate both liquids and solids and are dishwasher safe. After testing different measuring spoons, we settled on this set ourselves and used them in our kitchen every single day. Highly recommended!

- Mixing Bowls

For mixing salad dressings, spice rubs, marinades, sauces, and even storing leftovers, a set of high-quality mixing bowls is a must.
This 9-piece mixing bowl set from Luminarc can be used to do pretty much anything and won't absorb stains and odors because it's made of glass. Plus, these bowls stack easily for simple storage.

- Colander

For draining pasta or washing vegetables and salad greens, a colander is an essential piece for your minimalist kitchen. This 5-quart stainless-steel colander Good Grips is well designed and has ergonomic non-slip handles and "feet" so it doesn't slip all over the place.

- Vegetable Peeler

A vegetable peeler can speed up your preparation time, whether you're using it to peel potatoes, carrots, or any other vegetables.

We love this pirahna "Y-Peeler" because it's so simple. No multi-tasking here, but this is a high-quality peeler that will stand the test of time. It's dishwasher safe and ergonomically designed, just like all of our other recommendations.

- Potato Masher

Although a potato masher is a great tool, it usually has a very inconvenient and bulky shape that makes closing your drawer difficult. We chose this flip potato masher from Prepara for a few important reasons.

First, it "flips," which means that it's not a bulky tool to store in a drawer like most potato mashers are. Second, it's of high-quality stainless steel (with no BPA) and is dishwasher safe for easy cleaning.

- Whisk

A whisk is often one of the most used items in your kitchen, so it's important to have one that's ergonomically made. This 9-inch whisk Good Grips fits great in hand and is perfect for whisking together salad dressings, sauces, eggs, desserts, and much more.

Plus, it's dishwasher safe, so you don't have to worry about the handle melting or to warp in the heat.

- Salad Spinner

A salad spinner is your best friend when it comes to having a crisp salad. To prevent your greens from going soggy, you'll need to dry them, and "spinning" them is by far the easiest way to do it.

This salad spinner can be used by simply pressing the button on the top. It's very easy and simple to operate and even features a brake and locking mechanism for easy storage.

- Grater

One thing we're against here at Mealime is inefficiency. So what does this mean, exactly? It meals choosing multi-purpose tools and avoiding single-purpose tools whenever possible. Instead of purchasing different types of graters, a zester, and a chiffonade, why not choose one tool that can do it all?

- Shears

For cutting up a whole chicken and other meats, to vegetables, to stripping herbs, to even cutting the stems off of flowers

They're extremely sharp, heavy-duty, and comfortable. The blades are even separate for easy cleaning.

- Citrus Juicer

Sometimes it's the seemingly insignificant tasks in the kitchen that provide way more hassle than they should. Juicing a lemon or lime is one of those tasks!

It's difficult to do, your hands get juice on them, and the seeds often fall into your food. That's all solved with this quality citrus juicer from Prepworks. This one includes printed measurements, so you know exactly how much juice you've squeezed. It fits lemons, limes, and oranges and makes squeezing juice a joy. Plus, it's dirt cheap!

- Garlic Press

We still have this garlic press from Kuhn Rikon but use it less than we used to. If you don't like playing with garlic, and want the quickest solution, pick up this highly rated garlic press, and you'll be good to go. But if you don't mind crushing and chopping your garlic, you may want to pass on this item.

We've gone back and forth with garlic presses over the years and are currently on the "non-essential" train. A garlic press is nice to have and does make crushing garlic easier. But it's not that difficult to cut/press your garlic with just your chef's knife, and it's oddly satisfying to do so as well.

- Paring Knife

A paring knife is a kitchen knife with a short blade that can be used for many tasks. You can peel and chop with it, and the small tip is great for fine work like coring strawberries (or similar)

- Bread Knife

A bread knife is a serrated knife typically used for (wait for it...) slicing bread. A high-quality bread knife can also be used for slicing delicate items like cakes or pastry's.

- Honing / Sharpening Ceramic Rod

If you're going to purchase a quality chef's knife (which you should), you'll want to take care of it, so it lasts a lifetime. It doesn't take many tools or much time to maintain a quality knife, and this 12-inch ceramic honing rod from Messermeister is one of those tools.

Contrary to popular belief, most honing rods don't sharpen your blade. Rather, they realign your knife's edges quickly and efficiently. Because this honing rod is made of hard ceramic, it can both sharpen and honor your knives.

- Stainless Steel Skillet

A stainless steel skillet will likely be the workhorse of your kitchen. You will be using this cookware for frying, searing, sautéing, and browning, among other functions. For this reason, it's important to pick a high-quality stainless steel skillet that you can use for a lifetime.

- Sauté Pan

A saute pan is different from a skillet in a couple of important ways. It has a wide flat bottom and vertical sides that generally go up much higher than a skillet's flared sides do. This makes it easier to cook sauces and sear and braise meat than a skillet.

- Small Saucepan

A lightweight and easy to handle saucepan is necessary for small portion cooking of soups, stews, pasta, or sauces.

- Large Pot

You'll need a large pot to handle the volume for cooking large dishes like soups, stews, pasta, or sauces. They're extremely durable and cook evenly, thanks to their solid stainless steel and aluminum construction.

This large pot is perfect for cooking pasta, large dishes, or even making your broth.

- Cast Iron Skillet

Cast iron skillets have been workhorses in kitchens all over the world for over 2,000 years. Modern cast iron skillets are made from heavy cast iron and pre-seasoned (so food doesn't stick); with impressive heat retention abilities, these skillets are favored for use on both the stovetop and oven alike.

- Grill Pan

Grill pans have gained popularity in recent years. And why not? They're great for those without a barbecue (or who don't want to grill outside in the winter) but who still want those nice grill marks on their food.

For summer dishes like burgers, roasted salmon, meatballs, and marinated vegetables, a grill pan is necessary. It creates compelling grill lines in your food, just like a barbecue does. But it's much easier than barbecuing because you don't have to leave the comfort of your kitchen, and it only requires a stovetop element - no propane, gas, charcoal, or intense cleaning necessary.

- Baking Sheet Pan

A baking sheet pan (or sheet pan, baking tray, baking sheet) is a flat, rectangular metal pan used for roasting and baking food in the oven. From quickly roasting cauliflower, broccoli, or squash to whipping up a tasty treat if you're inclined to bake, a high-quality baking sheet pan is an essential item for a minimalist kitchen.

- Muffin Pan

A muffin pan is a baking pan with 6 or 12 built-in cups. Besides making muffins, they are great for individual quiches and on-the-go breakfast cups.

- Casserole Dish

A casserole dish is a large, deep dish with high edges used for baking or serving. For those lazy times, you want to throw a one-dish meal into the oven (like lasagna or a casserole), a quality casserole dish is a must.

- Broiler Pan

A broiler pan is a rectangular metal pan for use under the high-heat broiler in the oven. It is much thicker than a typical baking sheet pan, so it doesn't warp under the high heat and contains grooves and a draining pan that sits below to catch any fat that drips through (so your oven doesn't get stained).
Broiling is great when you want your food to get a nice brown crusty top.

- Stockpot

A stockpot is a very large pot (usually 12 quarts) that is ideal for homemade broth or large portions of soups. Anytime you want to make an extra-large meal is also a great reason to use a stockpot. But because most cooks don't tend to make their broth (though they should, it's easy!), this is not an essential item for a minimalist kitchen.

- Spatula

A spatula is a small cooking implement with a wide, flat, flexible blade used to mix, spread, and turn.
You may not think that a spatula can be much improved upon, but you'd be wrong! Tovolo has done a wonderful job with its line of stainless steel and silicon cooking implements.

- Slotted Spoon

This large spoon, featuring slots or holes for draining liquid, helps make cooking easier and safer. It is perfect to use when removing something from a pan while leaving the yummy juices behind.

- Tongs

For easily flipping meats and vegetables, a good pair of tongs that can handle all kinds of different sized foods is a must. They need to have silicone tips to prevent scratching and a high degree of heat-resistance to don't melt away after frequent use.

- Ladle

A ladle is essentially a very large, long-handled spoon. It is used for serving liquid dishes like soups, stews, or sauces.

- Oven Mitts

Oven mitts are used to protect your hands from being burned when transferring hot food to and from the oven. No longer will you have to wrap your hand in a tea towel and try not to spill your dish (or get burned) as you pull it out one-handed.

- Trivet

A trivet is a heat resistant pad that you place hot dishes on so you don't burn your table.

- Splatter Guard

A splatter guard is a device that is placed on top of skillets or sautés pans during high heat cooking to stop splattering hot oil and food from coating your stovetop.

- Thermometer

A quality meat thermometer is a must if you often cook meats and want to stop guessing at when they're done.

- Immersion Blender

An immersion blender (also known as a stick blender) is used to blend or puree food in the container it is being prepared in.

We use our immersion blender all the time. From blending soups and sauces directly in the pot to whipping up homemade whipped cream for dessert, to easily making mayonnaise for hard-boiled eggs,

- Kitchen Scale

For precisely measuring raw food (and coffee beans, in my case), a small, lightweight scale is needed.

- Blender

If you're a fan of making smoothies, sauces, dips, or soups, you'll likely want a powerful blender instead of using a food processor every time.

- Food Storage Containers

High-quality food storage containers are essential for bringing lunch to work and storing ingredients (or cooked meals) in the refrigerator, so they stay fresh for several days.

CHAPTER 6
Preparation Techniques

Techniques are a set of methods and procedures for preparing, cooking, and presenting food. Good techniques also take into account the economical use of food and cooking fuel resources and food safety.

The techniques used in preparing a dish can affect the dish as much if not more than the ingredients themselves. For this reason, many cooks believe it is more important to learn cooking techniques than to learn to follow recipes, as knowing a certain technique can improve a recipe or rescue one that has gone wrong.

Preparation Techniques

The techniqes used in preparing a dish can affect the dish as much if not more than the ingredients themselves. For this reason, many cooks believe it is more important to learn cooking techniques than to learn to follow recipes, as knowing a certain technique can improve a recipe or rescue one that has gone wrong. Here are the most basic cooking techniques to help you survive your first culinary year as a university student.

- Baking

This involves applying a dry convection heat to your food in an enclosed environment. The dry heat involved in the baking process makes the outside of the food go brown and keeps the moisture locked.

Baking is regularly used for cooking pastries, bread, and desserts.

- Frying

This means cooking your food in fat – there are several variations of frying:
- Deep-frying, where the food is completely immersed in hot oil
- Stir-frying, where you fry the food very quickly on high heat in an oiled pan
- Pan-frying, where food is cooked in a frying pan with oil; and
- Sauteing, where the food is browned on one side and then the other with a small quantity of fat or oil.

Frying is one of the quickest ways to cook food, with temperatures typically reaching between 175 – 225ºC.

- Roasting

Roasting is a high heat form of baking, where your food gets drier and browner on the outside by initial exposure to a temperature of over 500F. This prevents most of the moisture from being cooked out of the food. The temperature is then lowered to between 425 and 450F to cook through the meat or vegetables.

- Grilling

This is a fast, dry, and very hot way of cooking, where the food is placed under intense radiant heat. You can use various heat sources for grilling: wood-burning, coals, gas flame, or electric heating.

Before grilling, food can be marinated or seasoned.

A similar grilling method is broiling, where the heat source originates from the top instead of the bottom.

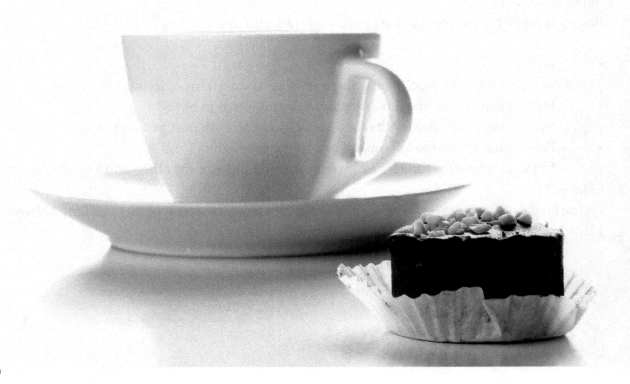

- Steaming

This means cooking your food in water vapor over boiling water. For this, it's handy to have a steamer, which consists of a vessel with a perforated bottom placed on top of another containing water.

Steam rises as the water boils, cooking the food in the perforated vessel above.

- Poaching

This involves a small amount of hot liquid, ideally at a temperature between 160 and 180F. The cooking liquid is normally water, but you can also use broth, stock, milk, or juice.

Common foods cooked by poaching include fish, eggs, and fruit.

- Simmering

This involves cooking liquid on top of a stove in a pot or pan. It should be carried out on low heat, and you will see bubbles appearing on the surface of the liquid as your dish cooks.

- Broiling

Similar to grilling, the heat source comes directly from the top. You should adjust your oven setting to broiling, but be careful, as this cooking method works quickly and your meal could easily become burned.

Favorite dishes for broiling include chicken, beef, and fish.

- Blanching

Here the food is part-cooked and then immediately submerged in ice-cold water to stop the cooking process.

All sorts of vegetables can be blanched, including green beans, asparagus, and potatoes.

- Braising

First, the food is sauteed or seared and then simmered in liquid for a long period until tender. Pot roasts, stews, and casseroles can be cooked in this way if they contain larger food items such as poultry legs.

- Stewing

Again, the food is sauteed or seared first, and then cooked in liquid, but normally uses smaller ingredients such as chopped meats or vegetables.

CHAPTER 7
Big Breakfast And Small Breakfast

We frequently hear the adage, "breakfast is the most important meal of the day." But is it? Or is that just a slogan cereal companies coined back in the 50s to sell more boxes? Does the size of your breakfast matter? And is skipping BreakfastBreakfast that bad?

As it turns out, whether and how you eat BreakfastBreakfast does have a big impact on your weight, focus, long-term health, and mood.

- A Big Breakfast Has Loads of Benefits

Eating a big breakfast has some obvious benefits. If you eat high-quality food, you're loading up your body with plenty of good fuel to take on the day. A good breakfast will keep your metabolism up, which is a necessity for athletes and students. Since a slow metabolism limits your ability to burn calories, it can lead to lower energy levels and hinder both your focus and endurance.

But a breakfast full of low-quality foods—such as pastries or sugar-filled cereals—simply packs on bad calories and will inevitably lead to a mid-morning crash. So it isn't just a big breakfast that's beneficial, but a big, healthy breakfast, full of fruit, whole grains, and lean proteins.

Eating a big breakfast confers amazing benefits when subsequent meals throughout the day—particularly dinner—are smaller in calories.

An isocaloric weight loss diet with exchanged caloric intake between BreakfastBreakfast and dinner differentially influences weight loss, waist circumference, serum ghrelin and lipids, appetite scores, and insulin resistance indices in overweight and obese women with the metabolic syndrome," the study concluded.

The extra weight loss might be a bit surprising, but the fact that the large-breakfast group was less hungry throughout the day isn't shocking. "Consuming a big breakfast in the morning, especially one including protein, fat, and fiber, can increase satiety throughout the day,

- A Small Breakfast Has Its Place

If an early morning workout prevents you from eating a big breakfast, Bonci suggests breaking up your meal into two parts—pre-workout and post-workout. That way, you'll have something in the tank for your workout without feeling weighed down, and you'll consume nutrients immediately after your workout, which can benefit recovery and muscle growth.

Forcing down a big breakfast before training won't do you much good if it ends up in the trashcan halfway through your workout. "If you're going to be doing an intense workout early in the day, you may want to rethink eating a big breakfast before. Too much food could result in an out-of-body experience!" Bonci says.

If you truly are someone who doesn't like to eat in the morning, forcing yourself to eat a big breakfast could leave you feeling lethargic—the exact opposite of what you want from your BreakfastBreakfast. If you find that a big breakfast doesn't work for you, try to break your BreakfastBreakfast up throughout the morning.

- No Breakfast Is A Big Mistake

Everyone's guilty of skipping BreakfastBreakfast now and then. Maybe you don't like to wake up early, maybe you're just not hungry, or maybe you think it will help you lose a few pounds. But skipping BreakfastBreakfast altogether is a bad move.

"BreakfastBreakfast is a way to get your fluid, fi ber, and protein quota for the day. "Without it, you're shortchanging your body and your mind. You'll be tired and have more trouble focusing."

Besides making you feel sluggish and cranky, skipping BreakfastBreakfast could have some insidious ramifications. A 2013 study from the Harvard School of Public Health found that "men who skipped breakfast had a 27% higher risk of CHD [coronary heart disease] compared with men who did not."

Though it sounds counterintuitive, missing BreakfastBreakfast might also lead to weight gain. A 2003 study found that "subjects who regularly skipped breakfast had 4.5 times the risk of obesity as those who regularly consumed breakfast." In this study, regularly skipping BreakfastBreakfast was defined as not eating Breakfast 75 percent of the time, and regularly eating BreakfastBreakfast was defined as eating it 95 percent of the time.

If you're an athlete or fitness-minded person who wants to live a healthy, high-performing lifestyle, skipping BreakfastBreakfast is not something you should do regularly. If you have a hard time eating Breakfast, Bonci suggests using your blender. She says, "If you truly don't have time or just don't have much of an A.M. appetite, how about BreakfastBreakfast in a blender? A smoothie or a shake can be an easy and convenient way to get something into your body."

CHAPTER 8
Breakfast

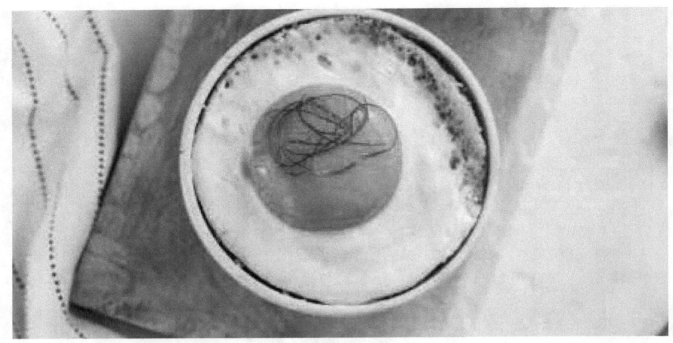

Egg & Bacon

PANCAKE BREAKFAST

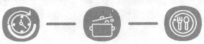

TIME
40

METHOD
EASY

SERVE
4

Directions:

Step 1

Whisk flour, baking soda, and 1/4 teaspoon salt in a medium bowl. Whisk milk, 1 egg, and oil in a small bowl. Add the milk mixture to the dry ingredients and whisk until smooth.

Step 2

Coat a medium nonstick skillet with cooking spray; heat over medium heat. Spoon 1/3 cup batter into the center of the pan. Immediately tilt and rotate the pan to spread the batter evenly over the bottom. Cook until the underside is golden brown, 1 1/2 to 2 minutes. Using a heatproof silicone or rubber spatula, lift the edge, quickly

Ingredients:

- ¾ cup white whole-wheat flour
- 1 ½ teaspoons baking soda
- ¼ teaspoon salt plus a pinch, divided
- 1 ½ cups reduced-fat milk
- 2 large eggs, divided
- 1 ½ tablespoon extra-virgin olive oil
- ⅛ teaspoon ground pepper
- 2 teaspoons minced fresh chives (optional)
- 1 slice bacon, cooked
- 1 teaspoon pure maple syrup

grab the pancake with your fingers and flip it over. Cook until the second side is golden brown, about 1 minute more. Slide onto a plate. Repeat with the remaining batter, spraying the pan as needed and stacking pancakes as you go to make 8 pancakes total.

Step 3

Wipe out the skillet and lightly coat it with cooking spray; heat over medium heat. Whisk the remaining egg, the remaining pinch of salt, PepperPepper, and chives (if using) in a small bowl. Pour into the pan and cook, gently stirring, until set, 2 to 3 minutes.

Step 4

To assemble a wrap:

Layer the egg across the bottom third of 1 warm pancake.

Top with bacon, drizzle with syrup, and roll-up.

Save the remaining pancakes for another time.

Tips

To make ahead: Refrigerate extra pancakes between wax paper sheets for up to 2 days or freeze for up to 1 month.

Nutrition Facts

Serving Size: 1 Wrap

Per Serving:

411 calories; protein 14.3g; carbohydrates 19.1g; dietary fiber 1.6g; fat 31.1g; saturated fat 5.2g; cholesterol 230.7mg; vitamin a iu 435.5IU; vitamin c 0.1mg; folate 30.7mcg; calcium 114.9mg; iron 3.2mg; magnesium 18.3mg; potassium 249.1mg; sodium 685.3mg; thiamin 0.1mg.

Exchanges:

4 Fat, 1 Medium-Fat Protein, 1 Starch, 1/2 High-Fat Protein, 1/2 Other Carbohydrate

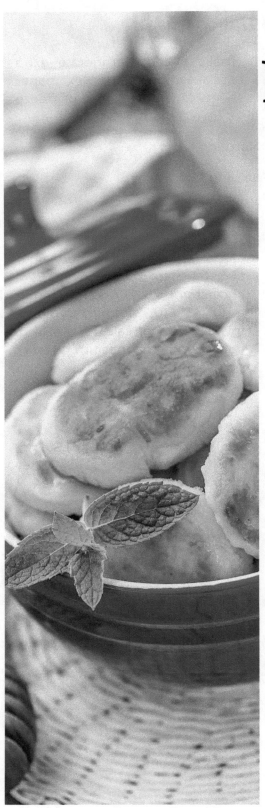

Grilled Cheese
PANCAKES

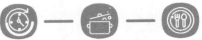

TOTAL TIME	PREP TIME	SERVE
35 MINS	15 MINS	4

Ingredients:

- 1 1/2 c. all-purpose flour
- 2 tsp. baking powder
- 1 tsp. kosher salt
- 1 tbsp. granulated sugar
- 1 c. plus 2 tbsp. milk
- 1/4 c. sour cream
- 1 large egg
- 3 tbsp. melted butter, plus more for pan
- 1 c. shredded cheddar
- 1 c. shredded mozzarella
- 1/4 c. freshly grated Parmesan
- Coarsely ground black PepperPepper
- 2 tbsp. mayonnaise
- Maple syrup, for serving

Directions:

Step 1

In a large bowl, whisk together flour, baking powder, salt, and sugar. In a medium bowl, whisk to combine milk, sour cream, egg, and melted butter. Gently fold dry ingredients into wet ingredients until just combined.

Step 2

In a large skillet over medium heat, melt ½ tablespoon butter. Pour a scant ⅓ cup pancake batter into the pan twice to make two pancakes. When little bubbles appear, about 3 to 4 minutes, flip one pancake and top with ¼ cup cheddar, ¼ cup mozzarella, 1 tablespoon Parmesan, and a pinch black pepper. Flip remaining pancake. Continue cooking until the second side is golden and cheese is melty, 3 minutes more.

Step 3

Top cheesy pancake with plain pancake, then evenly spread ½ tablespoon mayonnaise onto the top pancake. Flip and cook until a golden crust forms, 1 minute. Spread ½ tablespoon mayonnaise on to the second side, then flip to cook until a golden crust forms, 1 minute more. Transfer sandwich to a plate.

Step 4

Repeat with remaining batter, cheeses, and mayonnaise.

Step 5

Serve with maple syrup and garnish with bacon, if desired.

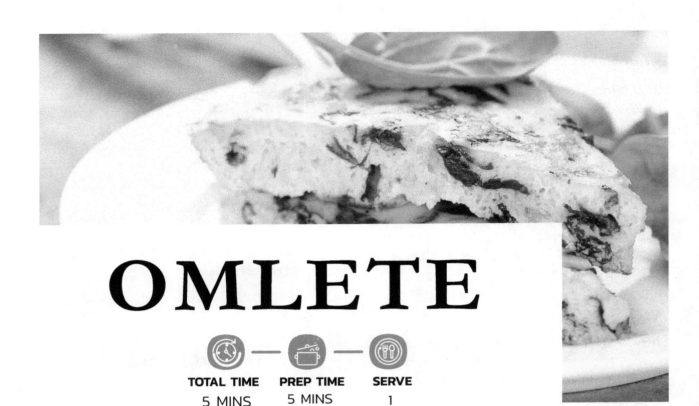

OMLETE

TOTAL TIME
5 MINS

PREP TIME
5 MINS

SERVE
1

Directions:

Step 1

Season the beaten eggs well with salt and Pepper. Heat the oil and butter in a nonstick frying pan over medium-low heat until the butter has melted and foamed.

Step 2

Pour the eggs into the pan, tilt the pan ever so slightly from one side to another to allow the eggs to swirl, and completely cover the pan's surface. Let the mixture cook for about 20 seconds, then scrape a line through the middle with a spatula.

Ingredients:

- 3 eggs, beaten
- 1 tsp sunflower oil
- 1 tsp butter

Step 3

Tilt the pan again to allow it to fill back up with the runny egg. Repeat once or twice more until the egg has just set.

Step 4

At this point, you can fill the omelet with whatever you like – some grated cheese, sliced ham, fresh herbs, sautéed mushrooms, or smoked salmon all work well. Scatter the filling over the top of the omelet and fold gently in half with the spatula. Slide onto a plate to serve.

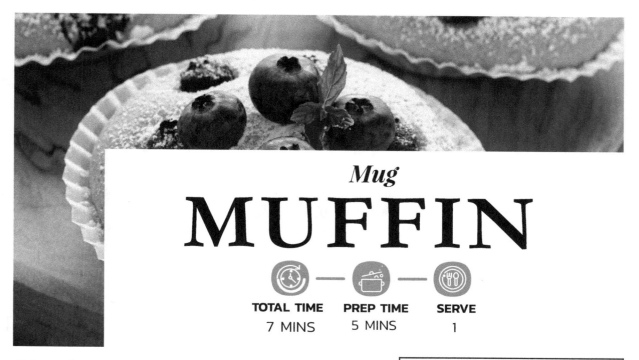

Mug
MUFFIN

TOTAL TIME 7 MINS — **PREP TIME** 5 MINS — **SERVE** 1

Directions:

Step 1

In a microwave-safe mug, stir together the flour, brown sugar, baking powder, salt, and cinnamon until well mixed.

Step 2

Add the butter to the mug and use your fingers to rub or smoosh them together until no large chunks of butter remain, and the mixture looks like damp sand (see photos below).

Step 3

Stir the milk into the butter/flour mixture. It should now resemble a thick muffin batter. If it's too dry, add a splash more milk. Sprinkle blueberries over the top and push them down into the batter. Microwave on high for approximately 90 seconds. Enjoy with a drizzle of maple syrup over the top.

Ingredients:

- 1/4 cup flour
- 1 Tbsp brown sugar
- 1/4 tsp baking powder
- 1/8 tsp salt
- pinch cinnamon
- 1/2 Tbsp butter
- 2 Tbsp milk
- 1-2 Tbsp frozen blueberries

Notes

Every microwave is different, so you may have to experiment with the exact cooking time.

You can add a drop or two of vanilla for extra flavor.

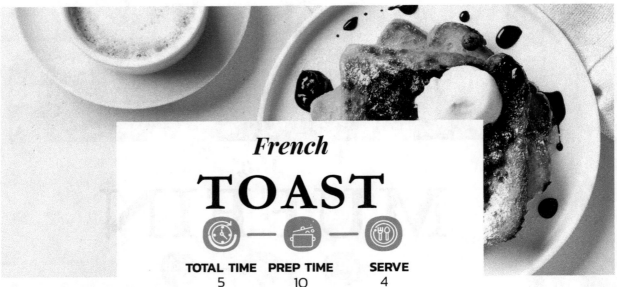

French
TOAST

TOTAL TIME	PREP TIME	SERVE
5	10	4

Directions:

Step 1

Whisk together eggs, milk, salt, sugar, vanilla, and cinnamon in a flat-bottomed pie plate or baking dish. Place bread slices, one or two at a time, into the egg mixture and flip to make sure both sides of bread are well-coated.

Step 2

Melt butter in a large skillet or on a griddle. Place bread slices in skillet or on the griddle and cook on medium heat until golden brown on each side, about 2-3 minutes.

Step 3

Serve immediately or keep warm in the oven until ready to serve, but no longer than about 30 minutes.

Nutrion Information

Calories: 225kcal | Carbohydrates: 32g | Protein: 9g | Fat: 5g | Saturated Fat: 2g | Cholesterol: 99mg | Sodium: 307mg | Potassium: 172mg | Fiber: 1g | Sugar: 10g | Vitamin A: 235IU | Calcium: 218mg | Iron: 2.2mg

Ingredients:

- 2 large eggs
- 1 cup milk, half and half, coconut milk, or almond milk
- pinch salt
- 1 tablespoon granulated sugar, honey, or maple syrup
- 1 teaspoon vanilla extract
- 1 teaspoon ground cinnamon
- 8 slices sandwich bread
- butter

Notes

You are simply dipping your bread slices into the egg mixture. If you leave your bread in the mixture for an extended amount of time, it will absorb more liquid and take longer to cook through.

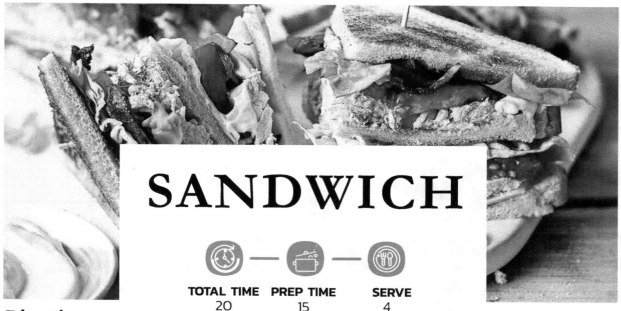

SANDWICH

TOTAL TIME	PREP TIME	SERVE
20	15	4

Directions:

Step 1

If using fresh Chicken (If not, skip to the next instruction) - Place chicken breasts into a saucepan, season with Salt and Pepper (or as desired), and pour enough water to cover it. Place over medium heat and bring to a boil. Cook until the chicken meat is tender.

Step 2

Transfer the chicken to a wide plate. If hot, allow it to cool, and shred the chicken meat with two forks. Transfer the chicken to a deep bowl, add the Mayonnaise, Ketchup, lemon juice, salt, and black PepperPepper to taste. Mix until everything is well blended and set aside.

Ingredients:

- 1/2 pound boneless Chicken
- 2 large Tomatoes Cut into slices
- 12 slices Pickles or as desired
- 9 slices Bread Toasted
- 3 Tbsp Mayonnaise
- 3 Tbsp Ketchup
- 1 Bunch Lettuce leaves
- 1 tbsp Lemon Juice
- Salt and PepperPepper to taste. To taste
- US Customary - Metric
- Get IngredientsPowered by Chicory

Step 3

Meanwhile, toast 9 slices of bread. Then, lay a slice of toast on a plate, or a board, add a thick layer of the chicken mixture on it, and cover it up with another layer of toast. Top this layer with about two Lettuce leaves, Pickles, and Tomato slices and cover it up with the third slice of toast.

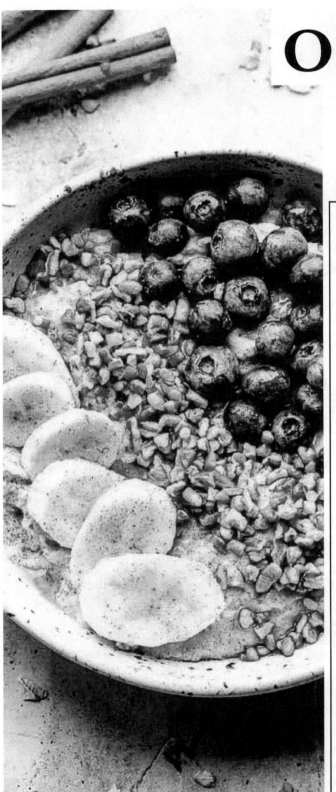

OATMEAL

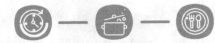

TOTAL TIME **PREP TIME** **SERVE**
2 MINS 4 MINS 1

Base Recipe

- ½ cup rolled old fashioned oats
- ½ cup milk of choice
- ½ cup of water
- Pinch of salt
- Maple Brown Sugar
- 1 teaspoon packed brown sugar
- 1 teaspoon maple syrup
- 2 tablespoons pecans chopped
- 1/8 teaspoon ground cinnamon

Banana Nut

- ½ banana sliced
- 2 tablespoons walnuts
- 1 tablespoon ground flaxseed
- 1/8 teaspoon ground cinnamon

Strawberry & Cream

- ½ cup sliced strawberries
- 1 tablespoon half and half
- 2 teaspoons honey
- 1/8 teaspoon vanilla extract

Strawberry & Cream

- 2 teaspoons cocoa powder
- 1 tablespoon peanut butter
- 2 teaspoons chocolate chips

Step 1

Place all the ingredients into a medium microwave-safe bowl and stir together. Heat in the microwave on high for 2 minutes. Then add 15-second increments until the oatmeal is puffed and softened. This is only necessary the first time you make it. Then you can gauge the exact time needed and repeat in the future. Stir before serving

Step 2

Stovetop Instructions

Step3

In a small saucepan, bring the water and milk to a boil. Reduce the heat to low and pour in the oats. Cook, occasionally stirring, until the oats are soft and have absorbed most of the liquid, about 5 minutes.

Step 4

Remove from the heat, cover, and let stand for 2-3 minutes.

Step 4

Assembly

Step 6

Stir in the toppings and let rest for a few minutes to cool. Thin with a little more milk, if desired. Serve warm.

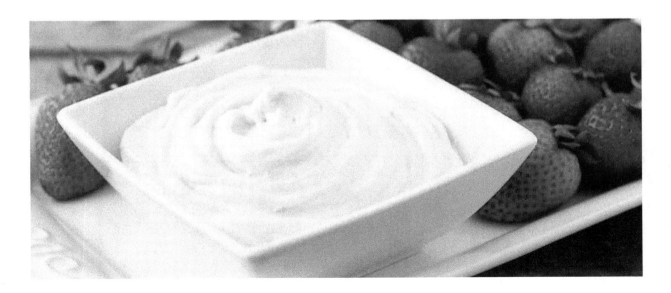

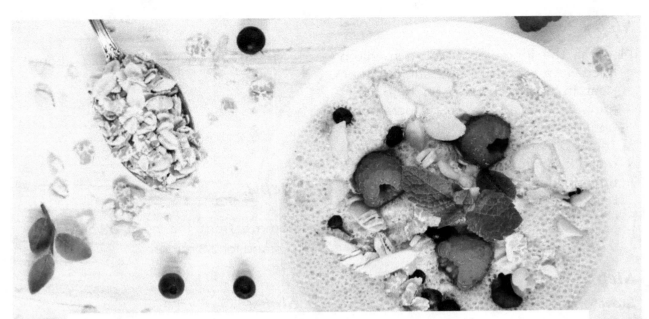

YOGURT

With Berries, Nuts, And Honey

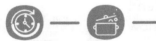

TOTAL TIME	PREP TIME	SERVE
5 MINS	5 MINS	1

Directions:

Step 1

Place yogurt in a dish, top with berries, nuts, and honey.

Step 2

Granola would taste great too.

Ingredients:

- 6 oz nonfat plain Greek yogurt
- 1 tbsp honey, local preferred
- 1/2 cup fresh berries
- 1 tbsp chopped walnuts

Nutrition

Calories: 250kcal, Carbohydrates: 35.5g, Protein: 19.5g, Fat: 4.5g, Saturated Fat: 0.5g, Sodium: 85.5mg, Fiber: 2.5g, Sugar: 31.

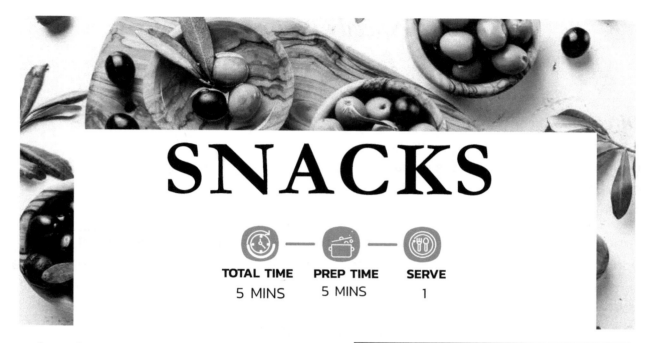

SNACKS

TOTAL TIME	PREP TIME	SERVE
5 MINS	5 MINS	1

Directions:

Step 1

Boil the pasta for 10-15 minutes, depending on the variety. The pasta should be soft and tender, not mushy or rubbery. Drain the water from the pasta.

Step 2

Stir in the sun-dried tomatoes. Pour in a dash of olive oil. Mix well. Top with a dash of salt and freshly ground black pepper.

Step 3

Serving Instructions, Variations, and Tips: Optional ingredient: Grated cheese can be sprinkled over the top of this dish immediately before serving. A few great pasta varieties for this recipe include whole wheat pasta, spelled or a gluten-free variety such as rice pasta or corn and millet pasta.

Ingredients:

- pasta snacks
- Pasta With Sun-dried Tomatoes
- Recipe Ingredients:
- 1 Box of pasta
- Jar of sun-dried tomatoes
- Olive oil
- Black PepperPepper
- Salt

Step 4

Cooking tip: Always allow the water to boil before you add the pasta. This prevents the pasta from getting soft and mushy. The saucepan can remain uncovered during the cooking process. Noodle pasta varieties tend to cook very quickly, so monitor closely. When finished, the pasta should be soft and tender but not mushy.

Speedy Pesto
PASTA

Directions:

Boil the pasta for 10-15 minutes, depending on pasta type.

Drain away the water from the pasta.

Stir in the pesto sauce.

Serving Instructions, Variations, and Tips: Optional

Ingredients:

- 1 Box of pasta
- Pesto sauce

ingredient: Sliced mushrooms can be stirred into the pasta right after it's finished cooking.

Optional ingredient: Grated garlic can be added and stirred into the pasta right before serving.

Remember that many pasta sauces include garlic, so you may want to skip this ingredient if you are using a sauce with garlic.

Creamy Oregano And
OLIVE PASTA

Ingredients:

- 1 Box of pasta
- Sliced olives
- Double cream
- Oregano
- Grated cheese

Directions:

Boil the pasta for approximately 10 to 15 minutes. The precise cooking time will vary according to pasta variety. It must be soft and tender.

Drain away the water.

Stir in the oregano, olives, and cream. Blend well.

Sprinkle grated cheese over top of the pasta immediately before serving.

Serving Instructions, Variations, and Tips: For a healthier snack, opt for organic cream for this recipe. Any variety of pasta will work for this recipe.

Make a gluten-free variation of this dish by using wheat-free pasta or another gluten-free variety of pasta. This simple pasta dish is quite filling, and it's appealing to most children, though some kids may prefer an olive-free version.

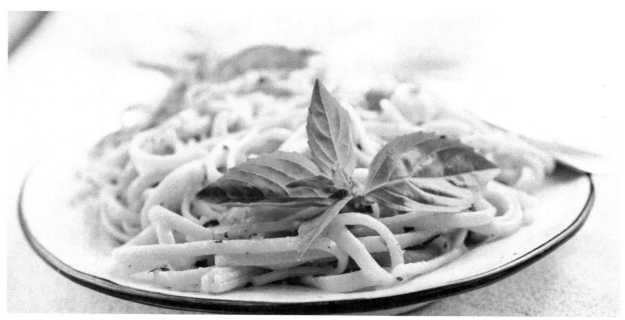

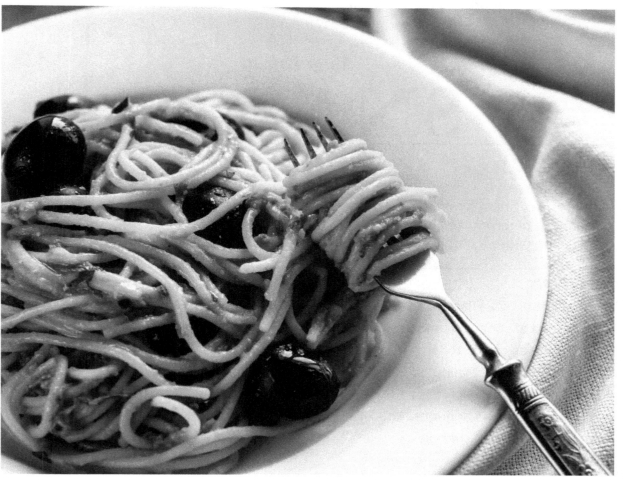

Tuna
PASTA

Directions:

Boil the pasta for approximately 10 to 15 minutes. The pasta must be soft and tender. Drain the water from the pasta Mix in the basil, tuna, and olive oil.

Sprinkle grated cheese on top or provide the cheese as a side when serving. Serving Instructions, Variations, and Tips: Add a bit of olive oil to this or any other pasta dish. The pasta with olive oil can make for a great snack when eaten alone. Optional ingredients: If desired, add salt and Pepper to taste. Any variety of pasta will work for this recipe. Make a gluten-free variation of this dish by using wheat-free pasta or another gluten-free variety of pasta.

Ingredients:

- 1 Box of pasta
- 1 Can of tuna
- Fresh basil
- (chopped)
- Grated cheese
- Olive oil

Vegetable
SNACKS

Ingredients:

- ¼ cup of onion (chopped)
- 1/2 cup of tomato (chopped)
- 1/2 cup of green PepperPepper
- (chopped)
- 1 cup of cheddar cheese (shredded)
- 4 8-inch soft tortillas

Directions:

Place the tortilla on a flat surface and sprinkle cheese over it.

Place chunks of chopped onions, green PepperPepper, and tomatoes over the cheese.

Fold the tortillas closed to form a half-circle.

Cook each tortilla for 2 minutes in a skillet over medium-high heat.

Flip the tortilla and cook for 1 additional minute.

Serving Instructions, Variations, And Tips:

Cut each tortilla into 4 triangles.

Serve with a salsa dip or sour cream.

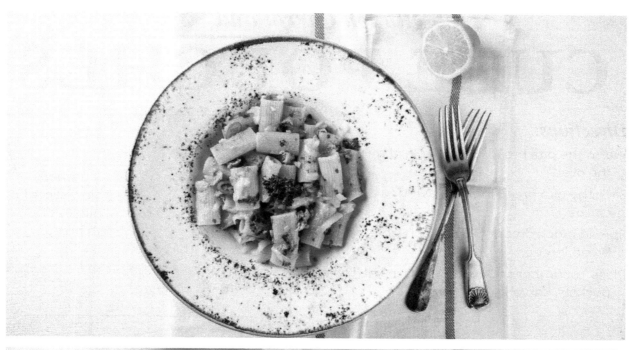

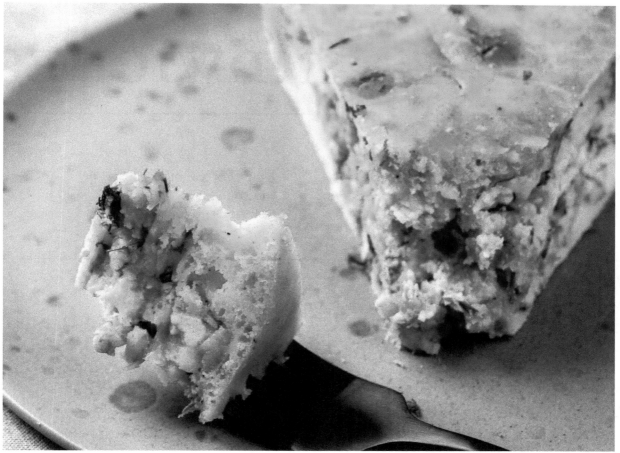

Ranch Carrot and
CUKE POUCHES

Directions:

Warm the pita bread for a couple of minutes in the oven.

Slice the pita bread in half, leaving two half-circles.

Spread ranch dressing onto each side of the pita bread interior.

Place cucumber and carrot slices inside the pita pockets. Serve!

Ingredients:

- 3 tablespoons of creamy ranch dressing
- 1 carrot (thinly sliced)
- 1 small cucumber (thinly sliced)
- 2 pieces of pita bread

Barbecue Ranch
VEGGIE SANDWICHES

Ingredients:

- 1 tablespoon of barbecue sauce
- 3 tablespoons of ranch salad dressing
- 2 large bun rolls
- 2 green pepper rings
- 2 slices of tomato
- 4 lettuce leaves
- 4 slices of cucumber

Directions:

Place the salad dressing and barbecue sauce in a mixing bowl and blend well.

Cut each bun in half. Apply the barbecue sauce and ranch dressing mix onto each bun half.

Place 2 lettuce leaves on each bun bottom. Add a tomato slice, a piece of PepperPepper, and 2 cucumber slices on top of the lettuce. Place the bun top on each sandwich and serve.

Serving Instructions, Variations, and Tips:

Opt for a salad dressing and barbecue sauce that's sugar-free and natural.

This dish makes a great after-school snack. Simply cut them into small bite-sized pieces.

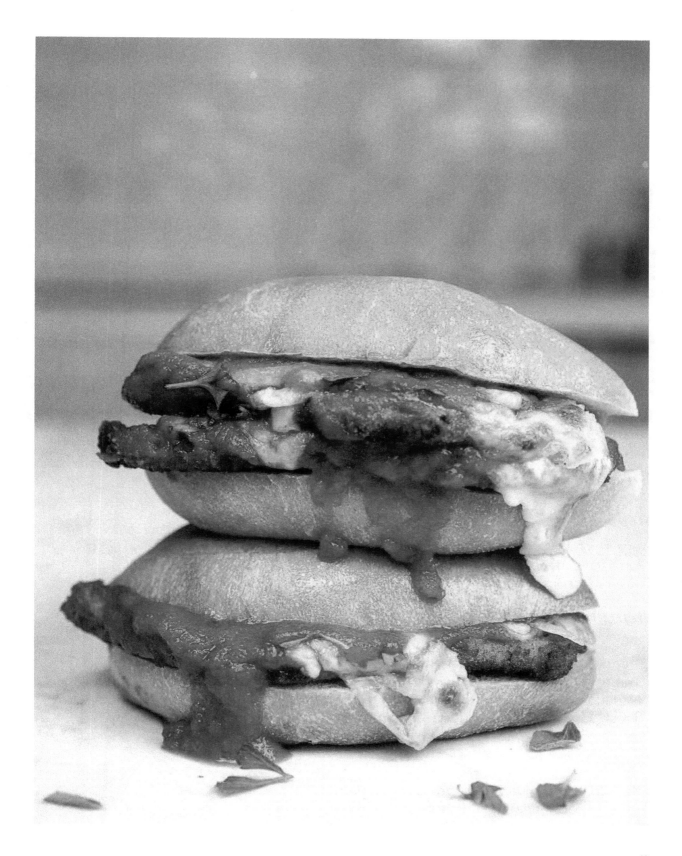

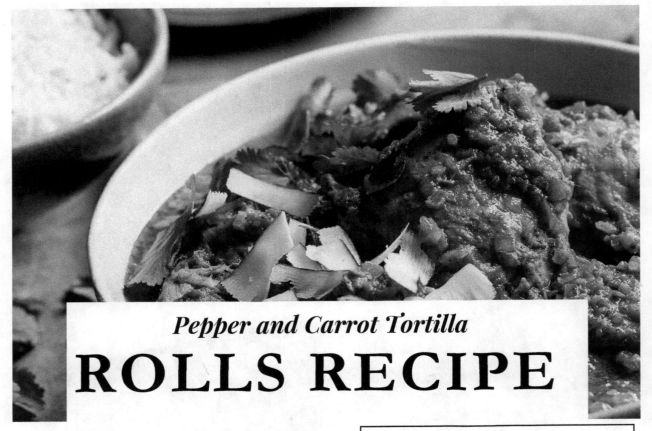

Pepper and Carrot Tortilla
ROLLS RECIPE

Directions:

Step 1

Warm the tortillas in the oven. Place each tortilla on a flat surface and coat each one with a thin layer of cream cheese.

Step 2

Sprinkle chunks of grated carrot and chopped PepperPepper over the cream cheese. Roll up the tortillas and serve. Serving Instructions, Variations, and Tips: Optional ingredients: Fresh spinach can be included in the rolls.

Step 2

If desired, opt for gluten-free tortillas or a gluten-free bread variety. Substitute the cream

Ingredients:

- 2 tablespoons of cream cheese
- 1 carrot (grated)
- 1 sweet red pepper (finely chopped)
- 2 soft flour tortillas

cheese with cottage cheese for a slightly different flavor.

CHAPTER 9
Bean Snacks

Speedy-Prep
BEAN STEW

Directions:

Mix the beans in a large bowl.

Add the tomato sauce and taco seasoning and blend well.

Heat and serve.

Serving Instructions, Variations, and Tips:

1.   This recipe makes approximately 6 servings.
2.   Whenever possible, opt for a sugar-free tomato sauce variety.

Ingredients:

- 1 can of hominy (canned)
- 1 can of kidney beans
- 1 can of pinto beans
- 1 can of garbanzo beans
- 6-ounces of tomato sauce
- 1 packet of taco seasoning

SPEEDY SPICY
Beans and Lentils

Ingredients:

- 1 can of lentils
- 1 can of pinto beans
- 1 can of garbanzo beans
- 1 can of kidney beans
- 1 can of great northern whites
- 1 can of French onion soup
- Salad Dressing
- Barbecue sauce

Directions:

Combine the lentils and beans in a large saucepan.

Add the soup to the lentils and beans.

Warm the ingredients over medium-low heat until it's thoroughly warmed.

Serving Instructions, Variations, and Tips:

Serve hot.

Add the dressing and sauce according to taste.

Opt for a low-fat dressing and barbecue sauce.

CHAPTER 9
Fruit Snacks

Cheese and
APPLE TOAST

Directions:

Mix the beans in a large bowl.

Add the tomato sauce and taco seasoning and blend well.

Heat and serve.

Serving Instructions, Variations, and Tips:
This recipe makes approximately 6 servings.

Whenever possible, opt for a sugar-free tomato sauce variety.

Ingredients:

- 1 1/2 cup apple sauce
- 4 slices of toast
- 4 slice of cheese
- Nutmeg

Cheese and Fruit
KEBAB RECIPES

Ingredients:

- 1 cup of grapes
- 1 cup of kiwi (cubed)
- 1 cup of apples (cubed)
- 1 cup of strawberries (quartered)
- 1-pound block of cheddar cheese (cubed)
- 4 skewers

Directions:

Alternate between cheese, kiwi, apple, cheese, strawberry, and grape onto each skewer.

Serving Instructions, Variations, and Tips: If desired, alternate between one fruit type and cheese on each skewer.

An array of other fruits and berries will work for this snack!

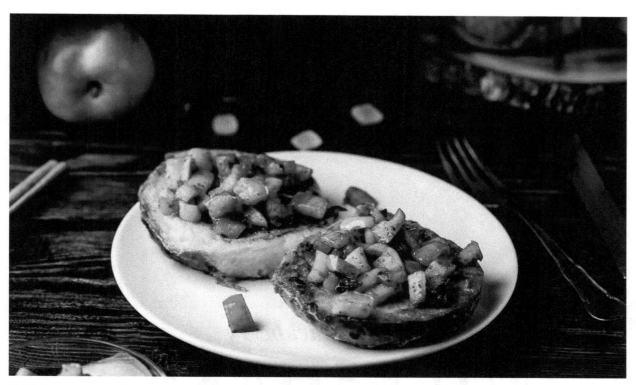

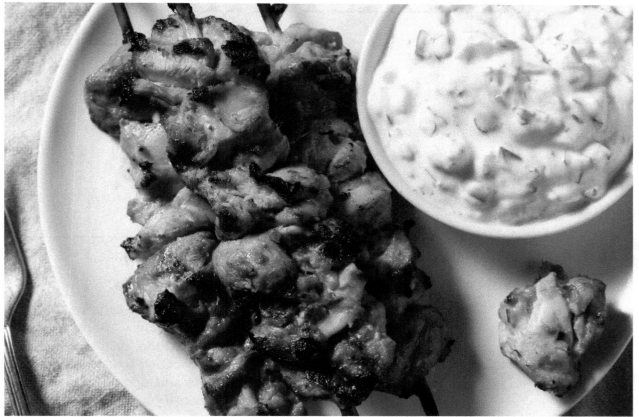

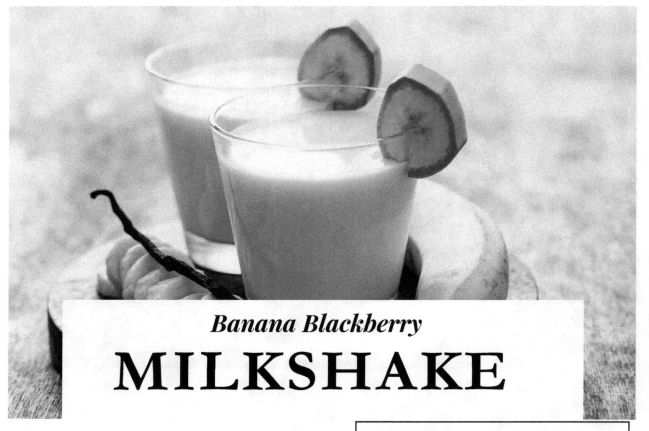

Banana Blackberry
MILKSHAKE

Directions:

Step 1

Pour the milk into a food processor or blender.

Step 2

Add the ice cubes, bananas, and blackberries

Step 3

Blend until the mixture is smooth and well-blended.

Step 4

Add the sugar substitute and blend momentarily to mix.

Ingredients:

- ¼ pint of fresh blackberries
- 1 pint of milk
- 1 banana (chopped)
- 6 ice cubes
- Sugar substitute
- Vanilla essence

Serving Instructions, Variations, and Tips:

Serve immediately. Use organic raw milk whenever possible. Popular sugar substitutes include xylitol, stevia, and honey. Remember that xylitol is very toxic to cats and dogs, so don't share with your pets if you use this ingredient

CHAPTER 9
Sandwich Snacks

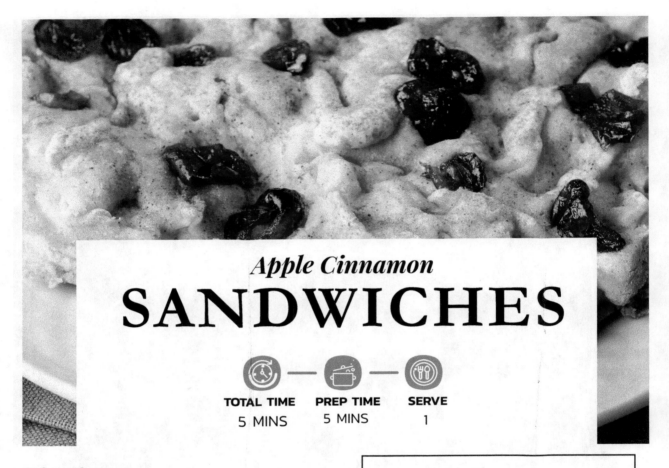

Apple Cinnamon
SANDWICHES

TOTAL TIME — **PREP TIME** — **SERVE**
5 MINS — 5 MINS — 1

Directions:

Step 1

Preheat your oven temperature on the grill or broil setting. Spread butter over the bread slices and lay them on an ungreased baking sheet.

Step 2

Add a few apple slices to the buttered bread. Sprinkle a bit of cinnamon over the apples.

Step 3

Broil or grill for approximately 2 minutes. They should be a pale golden brown color.

Ingredients:

- 1 tablespoon of butter
- 1 tablespoon of cinnamon
- 4 slices of apple bread
- 1 apple (peeled, core removed and sliced)

Serving Instructions, Variations, and Tips:

This recipe makes 4 servings. Consult the gluten-free bread section for the apple bread recipe!

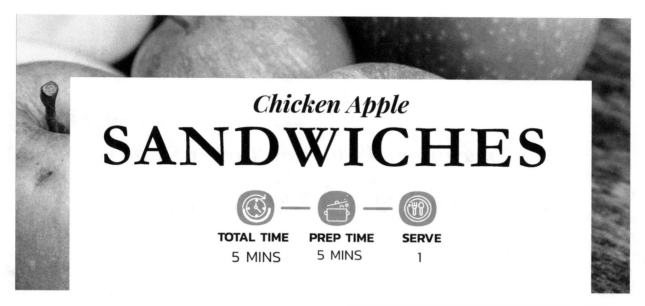

Chicken Apple
SANDWICHES

TOTAL TIME
5 MINS

PREP TIME
5 MINS

SERVE
1

Directions:

Step 1

Cut the chicken into bite-sized pieces. Chop the Braeburn apple into small, bite-sized chunks.

Step 2

Combine the lemon juice, ginger, and mayonnaise in a mixing bowl. Add the celery, apple, and chicken. Mix well.

Step 3

Slice the baguette. Place watercress on one side of the baguette and place the mix on the other side. Place onion on top and serve.

Ingredients:

- 1 teaspoon of fresh ginger-root (grated) 2 1/4 teaspoons of
- lemon juice
- 1/2 cup of mayonnaise
- 1 cup of cooked chicken
- 1 bunch of watercress
- 1 Braeburn apple
- 1 celery rib (chopped)
- 1 medium red onion (peeled and thinly sliced)
- 1 baguette

Serving Instructions, Variations, and Tips:

This recipe makes 4 servings. If desired, use basil or another herb in place of watercress.

Season to taste with salt and Pepper.

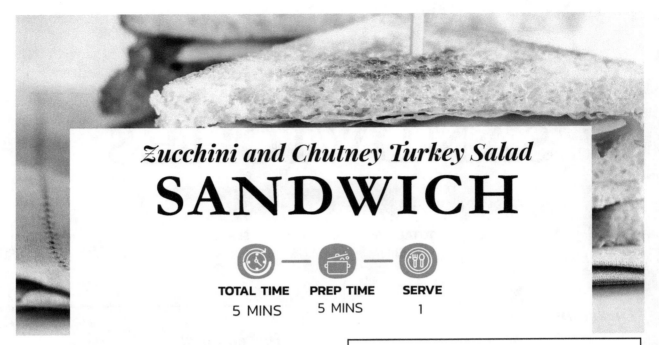

Zucchini and Chutney Turkey Salad
SANDWICH

TOTAL TIME
5 MINS

PREP TIME
5 MINS

SERVE
1

Directions:

Step 1

Preheat your oven to 350 degrees F. Cut the zucchini lengthwise into 1/4-inch wide slices. Place the turkey, mayonnaise, chutney, celery, and sesame seeds in a medium bowl and mix. Thoroughly coat the meat. Brush a bit of olive oil onto each piece of bread.

Step 2

Lay the bread (in 1 layer) onto a cookie sheet. Bake for approximately 12 minutes. The bread must be golden and lightly toasted. Apply a bit of turkey salad to 4 pieces of bread.

Step 3

Stack the peppers, spinach leaves, and zucchini on top of the turkey salad. Drip a bit of salad dressing over the veggies. Apply some mustard to the other 4 pieces of bread and top the veggies to complete the sandwiches.

Ingredients:

- 1 teaspoon of sesame seeds (toasted)
- 2 tablespoons of olive oil
- 2 tablespoons of Caesar dressing
- 3 tablespoons of mayonnaise
- 4 teaspoons of Dijon mustard
- 1/3 cup of hot mango chutney
- 1/2 cup of celery (finely chopped)
- 2 cups of cooked turkey (chopped into small pieces) 7-ounces of roasted red bell peppers (drained and sliced) 1 zucchini
- 8 spinach leaves

Serving Instructions, Variations, and Tips:

If desired, use ranch dressing or another favorite dressing variety. You can also use different veggies.

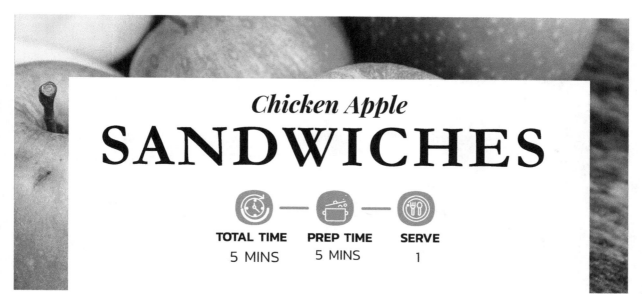

Chicken Apple
SANDWICHES

TOTAL TIME 5 MINS — **PREP TIME** 5 MINS — **SERVE** 1

Directions:

Step 1

Cut the chicken into bite-sized pieces. Chop the Braeburn apple into small, bite-sized chunks.

Step 2

Combine the lemon juice, ginger, and mayonnaise in a mixing bowl. Add the celery, apple, and chicken. Mix well.

Step 3

Slice the baguette. Place watercress on one side of the baguette and place the mix on the other side. Place onion on top and serve.

Ingredients:

- 1 teaspoon of fresh ginger-root (grated) 2 1/4 teaspoons of
- lemon juice
- 1/2 cup of mayonnaise
- 1 cup of cooked chicken
- 1 bunch of watercress
- 1 Braeburn apple
- 1 celery rib (chopped)
- 1 medium red onion (peeled and thinly sliced)
- 1 baguette

Serving Instructions, Variations, and Tips:

This recipe makes 4 servings. If desired, use basil or another herb in place of watercress.

Season to taste with salt and Pepper.

CHAPTER 10
Sauce

Cheese
SAUCE

Try this over broccoli or cauliflower. It's wonderful!

Directions:

In a heavy-bottomed saucepan over the lowest heat, warm the cream to just below a simmer.

Whisk in the cheese about 1 tablespoon at a time, only adding the next tablespoonful after the last one has melted. When all the cheese is melted in, whisk in the dry mustard, and serve.

Ingredients:

- 1/2 cup heavy cream
- 3/4 cup shredded Cheddar cheese
- 1/4 teaspoon dry mustard

Serving Instructions, Variations, and Tips:

Enough to sauce 1 pound of broccoli or cauliflower, or about 4 servings of sauce, each with 1 gram of carbohydrates, no fiber, and 6 grams of protein.

Stir-Fry
SAUCE

If you like Chinese food, make this up and keep it on hand. Then you can just throw any sort of meat and vegetables in your wok or skillet and have a meal in minutes.

Ingredients:

- 1/2 cup soy sauce
- 1/2 cup dry sherry
- 2 cloves garlic, crushed
- 2 tablespoons grated fresh ginger
- 2 teaspoons Splenda

Directions:

Combine the ingredients in a container with a tight-fitting lid, and refrigerate until you're ready to use.

Not-Very-Authentic
PEANUT SAUCE

This is inauthentic because I used substitutes for such traditional ingredients as lemongrass and fish sauce. I wanted a recipe that tasted good but could be made without a trip to a specialty grocery store.

Directions:

Put all the ingredients in a blender, and run it until everything is well combined and smooth. If you'd like it a little thinner, add another tablespoon of chicken broth.

Ingredients:

- 1 piece of fresh ginger about the size of a walnut, peeled and thinly sliced across the grain
- 1/2 cup natural peanut butter, creamy
- 1/2 cup chicken broth
- 1 1/2 teaspoons lemon juice
- 1 1/2 teaspoons soy sauce
- 1/4 teaspoon Tabasco sauce
- 1 large or 2 small cloves garlic, crushed
- 1 1/2 teaspoons Splenda

Serving Instructions, Variations, and Tips:

About 2 cups, or 16 servings, each with 2 grams of carbohydrates, a trace of fiber, and 2 grams of protein.

Hoisin
SAUCE

This Chinese sauce is usually made from fermented soybean paste, which has tons of sugar in it. Peanut butter is inauthentic, but it tastes quite good here.

Ingredients:

- 4 tablespoons soy sauce
- 2 tablespoons creamy natural peanut butter
- 2 tablespoons Splenda
- 2 teaspoons white vinegar
- 1 clove garlic, crushed
- 2 teaspoons toasted sesame oil
- 1/8 teaspoon Chinese Five Spice powder

Directions:

Put all the ingredients in a blender, and run it until everything is smooth and well, combined. Store in a snap-top container.

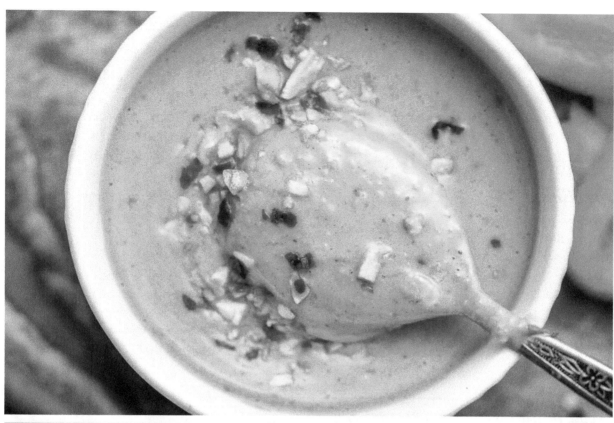

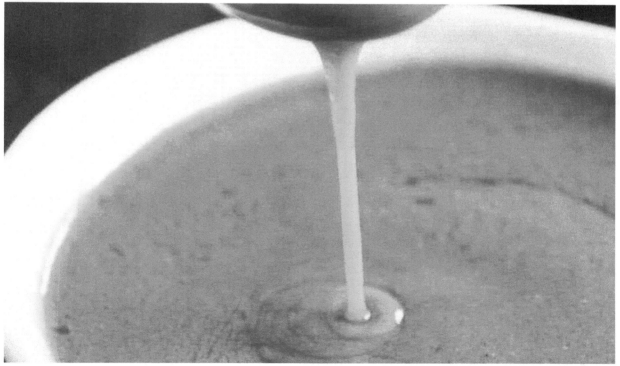

Taco
SEASONING

Many store-bought seasoning blends include sugar or cornstarch-my food counter book says that several popular brands have 5 grams of carbs in 2 teaspoons! This is low-carb, very easy to put together, tastes great, and it is even cheaper than the premixed stuff.

Directions:

Combine all the ingredients, blending well, and store in an airtight container. Use 2 tablespoons of this mixture to flavor 1 pound of ground beef, turkey, or chicken. .

Ingredients:

- 2 tablespoons chili powder
- 1 1/2 tablespoons cumin
- 1 1/2 tablespoons paprika
- 1 tablespoon onion powder
- 1 tablespoon garlic powder
- 1/8 to 1/4 teaspoon cayenne pepper (less makes a more mild seasoning, more takes the spice up a notch)

Serving Instructions, Variations, and Tips:
About 8 tablespoons, or 4 batches worth. 2 tablespoons will add just under 2 grams of carbohydrates to a 4-ounce serving of taco meat.

Chicken
SEASONING

This is wonderful sprinkled over the chicken before roasting.

Directions:

Combine all the ingredients well, and store in a salt shaker or the shaker from an the old container of herbs. Sprinkle over the chicken before roasting; I use it to season at the table, as well.

Ingredients:

- 3 tablespoons salt
- 1 teaspoon paprika
- 1 teaspoon onion powder
- 1 teaspoon garlic powder
- 1 teaspoon curry powder
- 1/2 teaspoon black pepper

Serving Instructions, Variations, and Tips:
Just over 1/4 cup. There are 7 grams of carb in this whole recipe and 1 gram of fiber, for a total of 6 grams of usable carbs, so the amount in the teaspoon or so you sprinkle over a piece of chicken is negligible.

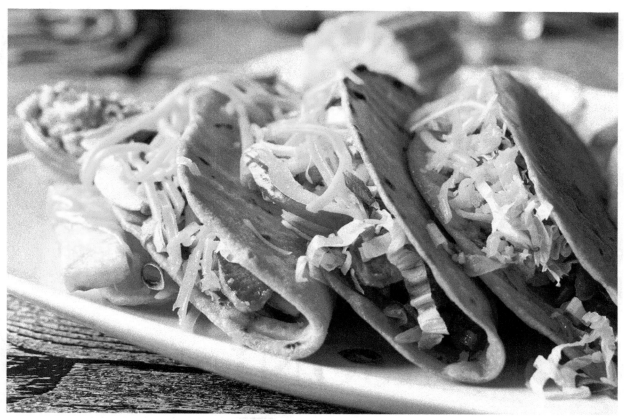

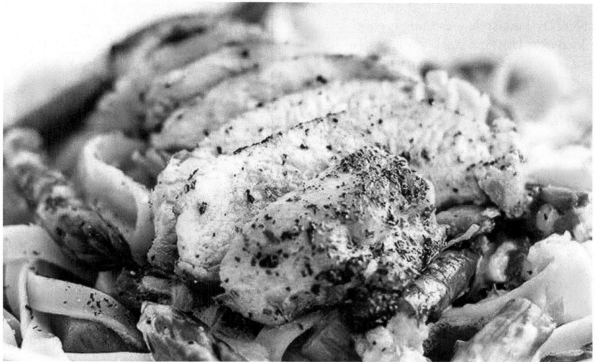

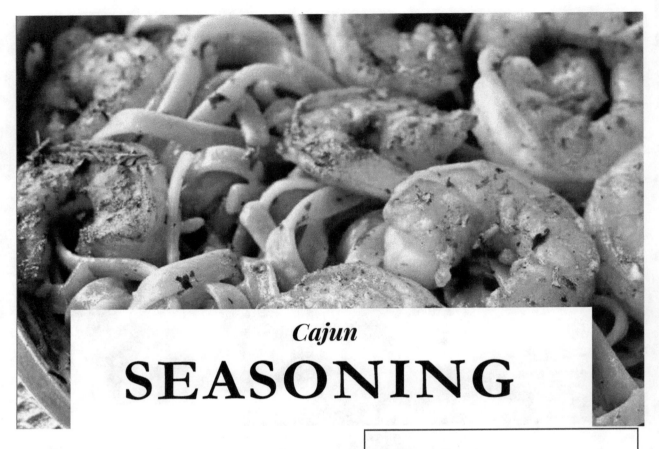

Cajun
SEASONING

This New Orleans-style seasoning is good sprinkled over chicken, steak, pork, fish, or just about anything else you care to try it on.

Directions:

Step 1

Combine all ingredients thoroughly, and store in an airtight container.

Ingredients:

- 2 1/2 tablespoons paprika
- 2 tablespoons salt
- 2 tablespoons garlic powder
- 1 tablespoon black pepper
- 1 tablespoon onion powder
- 1 tablespoon cayenne pepper
- 1 tablespoon dried oregano
- 1 tablespoon dried thyme

Serving Instructions, Variations, and Tips:

2/3 cup. In the entire batch, there are 37 grams of carbohydrates and 9 grams of fiber, for a total of 28 grams of usable carbs. Considering how spicy this is, you're unlikely to use more than a teaspoon or two at a time, and 1 teaspoon has just 1 gram of carbohydrates and a trace of fiber.

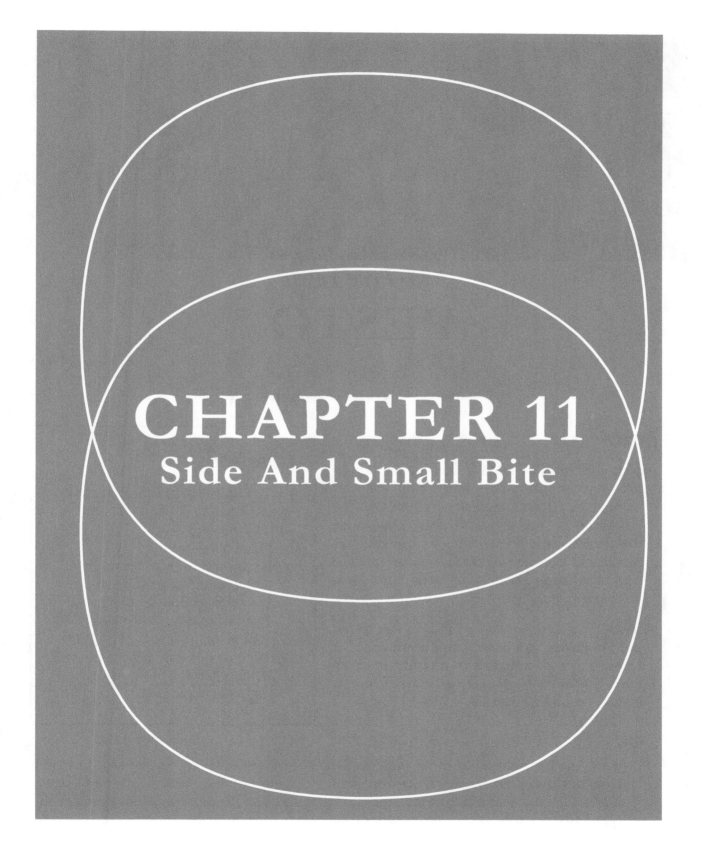

CHAPTER 11
Side And Small Bite

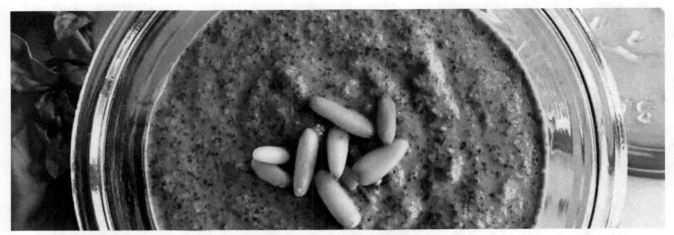

Nut-Free Vegan

PESTO

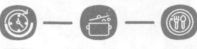

TIME
5

COOK
0

SERVE
1

Directions:

Blend: add the pumpkin seeds, garlic, lemon juice, nutritional yeast, basil, chili flakes if using, and salt to a food processor. Close the lid, begin to process, and then slowly use the device's opening to pour in the olive oil. Process for at least 60-90 seconds, or until the pumpkin seeds are finely chopped and have softened slightly.

Store & Serve: season with additional salt or red pepper flakes, if desired. Use immediately, or transfer to a container with a tight-fitting lid. Store in the fridge for up to 7 days or in the freezer for up to 2 months.

Ingredients:

- 1/3 cup (48 g) pumpkin seeds or pepitas
- 3 cloves of garlic
- Juice of 1 lemon*
- 3 tablespoons nutritional yeast
- 2 ounces (55 g) fresh basil, de-stemmed (about 2 cups)
- 1/2 teaspoon red chili flakes (optional)
- 1/2 teaspoon salt, or to taste
- 1/2 cup (120 ml) high-quality extra virgin olive oil

Notes

Pumpkin Seeds: there is no other nut-free substitute that I would recommend for this recipe, but pumpkin seeds can be replaced with pine nuts or walnuts. Lemon Juice: lemon juice adds some brightness and acidity to the dish. Because it's being used raw. It's best to use fresh, as the carton/canned substitutes are often less flavorful.

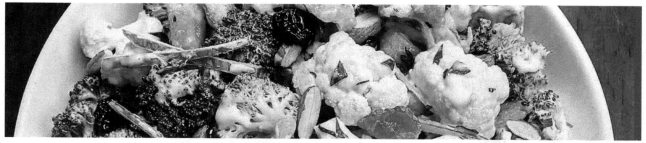

Marinated Cauliflower

SALAD

TIME	COOK	SERVE
45	15	8

Directions:

Make the dressing first, so the flavors have time to blend. In a jar or bowl, combine the olive oil, red wine vinegar, Dijon, garlic powder, Italian seasoning, salt, pepper, and Parmesan. Whisk the ingredients together or close the jar and shake until combined. Set the dressing aside.

Remove the leaves and stem from the cauliflower, then chop it into very small florets (about a grape's size). Place the chopped cauliflower in a large bowl. Drain the black olives and remove the banana peppers from the jar. Add both to the bowl with the cauliflower. Dice the red bell pepper and finely dice the red onion and parsley. Add them to the bowl. Pour the prepared dressing over the salad, then toss to combine. Refrigerate the salad for at least 30 minutes to allow the flavors to absorb. Stir again just before serving. This salad gets better as it refrigerates, and the cauliflower has more time to marinate. Always stir just before serving to redistribute the flavors.

Ingredients:

- ½ cup olive oil
- ¼ cup red wine vinegar
- 1 tsp Dijon mustard
- ¼ tsp garlic powder
- 1 Tbsp Italian seasoning
- ½ tsp salt
- ¼ tsp freshly cracked black pepper
- 2 Tbsp grated Parmesan
- Salad
- 1 head cauliflower
- 1 2.25oz. can sliced black olives
- ½ 12oz. jar banana pepper rings
- 1 red bell pepper
- ⅓ cup diced red onion
- 2 Tbsp chopped fresh parsley

Notes

Store-bought Italian dressing can be used in place of homemade. Nutrition Serving: 1cup ⊠ Calories: 175.66kcal ⊠ Carbohydrates: 8.06g ⊠ Protein: 2.69g ⊠ Fat: 15.6g ⊠ Sodium: 431.44mg ⊠ Fiber: 2.7g

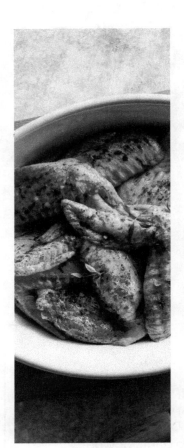

Garlic Marinated
CHICKEN

TOTAL TIME	COOK TIME	SERVE
1H	15 MINS	4

Ingredients:

- 1/4 cup olive oil
- 1/4 cup lemon juice
- 3 cloves garlic, minced
- 1/2 Tbsp dried oregano
- 1/2 tsp salt
- Freshly cracked pepper
- 1.5 lbs. boneless skinless chicken breasts

Directions:

the olive oil, lemon juice, garlic, oregano, salt, and pepper to a bowl or a large zip-top bag. Stir the ingredients in the dish until combined.

Filet each chicken breast into two thinner pieces. Place the pieces in the bag or a shallow dish, then pour the marinade over the top, making sure the chicken pieces are completely covered in marinade. Marinate the chicken for 30 minutes, or up to 8 hours (refrigerated), occasionally turning to maximize the chicken's contact with the marinade.

When ready to cook, heat a large skillet over medium. Transfer the chicken from the marinade to the hot skillet and cook on each side until well browned and cooked through (about 5-7 minutes each side, depending on the pieces' size). Cook two pieces to avoid overcrowding the skillet, which can cause juices to pool and prevents browning. Discard the excess marinade.

Transfer the cooked chicken from the skillet to a cutting board and rest for five minutes before slicing and serving.

Notes

*This marinade can also be used for chicken thighs. The amount of marinade listed in the recipe can handle about 4-6 chicken thighs, depending on their size.

Nutrition

Serving: 1Serving ⊠ Calories: 331.5kcal ⊠ Carbohydrates: 2.28g ⊠ Protein: 38.35g ⊠ Fat: 11.3g ⊠ Sodium: 432.18mg ⊠ Fiber: 0.4g

CHAPTER 12
Streetfood

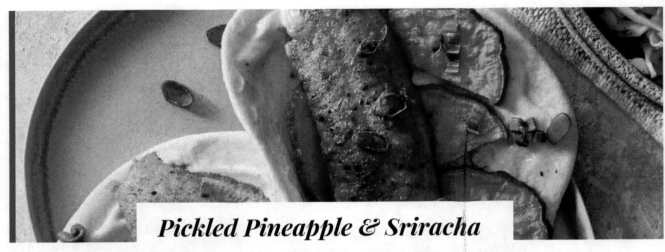

Pickled Pineapple & Sriracha

GRILLED CHEESE

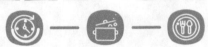

TIME	PREP TIME	SERVE
25	15	4

Directions:

Step 1

Bring all the pineapple pickle ingredients to a boil with 100ml water. Add the pineapple chunks and toss in the pickle. Allow to cool, then transfer to a bowl, cover with cling film

Step 2

Spread the sourdough slices with mayonnaise on one side. Put half the butter and the rapeseed oil in a frying pan over medium heat. When the butter has melted, put one slice of bread in the pan, mayo-side down, and top with a slice of cheddar, some spring onion, pickled pineapple, and more cheese and sriracha, to taste. Top with the other piece of bread, mayo-side up.

Step 3

Cook for about 3 mins or until crispy and golden underneath, then turn the sandwich over and add the rest of the butter. Cook until crisp and golden on that side, and the cheddar is melting. Slice in half and serve immediately.

Ingredients:

- ½ pineapple, flesh cut into small cubes
- 2 thick slices of sourdough
- 1 tbsp mayonnaise
- 1 tbsp unsalted butter
- 2 tsp rapeseed oil
- 85g cheddar, sliced
- 1 spring onion, finely sliced
- sriracha chili sauce
- 100ml white wine vinegar
- 40g golden caster sugar
- ½ tsp coriander seeds
- ½ tsp mustard seeds
- ½ tsp black peppercorns
- 1-star anise
- 1 bay leaf

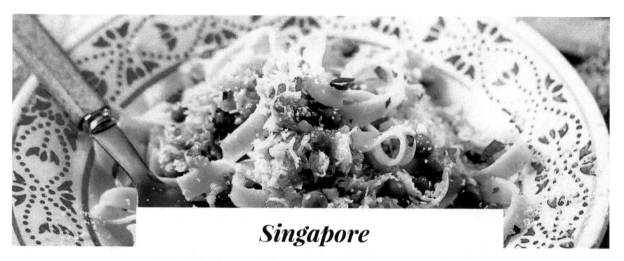

Singapore

CHILI CRAB

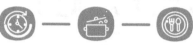

TIME	PREP TIME	SERVE
30	25	4

Directions:

Step 1

The crab must be prepared before stir-frying (you can ask your fishmonger to do this). This involves removing the claws, the main shell, discarding the dead man's fingers, then cutting the body into four pieces, and cracking the claws and the legs so the sauce can get through to the meat.

Step 2

Heat the oil in a large wok and sizzle the garlic, ginger, and chopped chilies for 1 min or until fragrant. Add the ketchup, soy, and 100ml water, and stir to combine. Throw in the crab, turn up the heat, and stir-fry for 3-5 mins or until the crab is piping hot and coated in the sauce. Stir through most of the coriander, spring onions, and sliced chili

Step 3

Use tongs to arrange the crab on a serving dish, pour over the sauce from the pan, and scatter over the remaining coriander, spring onions, and sliced chili. Serve with rice or bao buns and a lot of napkins.

Ingredients:

- 1 whole cooked crab (about 1kg)
- 2 tbsp flavorless oil
- 3 garlic cloves, very finely chopped thumb-sized piece ginger, very finely chopped
- 3 red chilies, 2 very finely chopped, 1 sliced
- 4 tbsp tomato ketchup
- 2 tbsp soy sauce
- handful coriander leaves, roughly chopped 2 spring onions, sliced
- rice or steamed bad buns, to serve

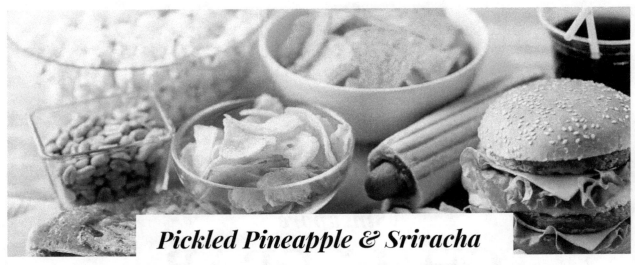

Pickled Pineapple & Sriracha

GRILLED CHEESE

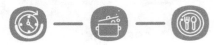

TIME	PREP TIME	SERVE
25	15	4

Ingredients:

- For the puris
- 150g chakki atta (chapatti flour)
- 30g fine semolina
- 1l vegetable oil, for puris and deep-frying
- For the pani (water)
- 50g bunch coriander
- 25g bunch mint
- 5g fresh ginger
- 2 green chilies
- 2 tbsp tamarind pulp

- 500ml chilled water
- 1 tsp ground cumin
- 2 tsp red chili flakes
- ¼ tsp asafoetida
- For the filling
- 400g canned chickpeas
- ¼ tsp asafoetida
- 2 large potatoes, peeled and diced into 1cm cubes
- 1 tsp ground cumin
- 1 medium red onion, finely chopped
- small bunch coriander including stalks, finely chopped
- juice of 1/2 lemon

Directions:

Step 1

Make the pani water. Place the coriander, mint, ginger, green chilies, and tamarind pulp in a blender and blitz into a paste. Place in a water jug and add the chilled water and remaining ingredients. Mix well and chill in the fridge for at least 2 hours.

Step 2

Begin making the puris. Combine the chakki atta, fine semolina, a little sea salt to season, and 1 tbsp of the vegetable oil in a large bowl. Mix well and then gradually add 80-85ml of luke-warm water to create a stiff dough. Cover with a clean damp tea towel and allow to rest for 30 mins.

Step 3

For the filling, place the chickpeas and potatoes in separate large pans. Cover both with water and add 1/4 tsp asafoetida to the chickpea pan. Bring broth to a boil. Cook the potatoes until softened and then drained. Once the chickpea pan is boiling, bring down to a simmer and cook for a further 10 mins. Drain both together and leave to cool.

Step 4

Once the dough has rested, grease your fingers with oil and knead the dough for at least 5 mins. Return the dough to the bowl, cover again and rest for a further 30 mins.

Step 5

Once rested, knead again with a little oil for a further 5 mins. You should now have a very smooth dough. Cover and allow to rest for a further 30 mins.

Step 6

Once the chickpeas and potatoes have cooled, please place them in a large bowl with the other filling ingredients, season, and mix well.

Step 7

Divide the dough into 3 and roll out 1/3 to 50p thickness and use a cookie cutter to cut disks 6cm in diameter. Cover the disks with a damp tea towel. Repeat with the other 2/3rds of the dough. Rest the disks for another 30 mins. Heat your oil to 180C (if you don't have a thermometer, simply take a tiny piece of bread, and if it turns golden brown in seconds, your oil is ready). Carefully place the puris into the oil, and when they begin to rise to the surface, gently hold a spoon down on top of them. This helps the puris to puff up. When the puris are golden brown, remove with a slotted spoon and drain on absorbent kitchen paper.

Step 8

To eat, take a crisp puri, create a small hole in the center. Fill the puri with a little of the chickpea and potato filling. Then pour in the chilled pan and finally add a little sev and a few fresh pomegranate seeds. Eat the puri in one go

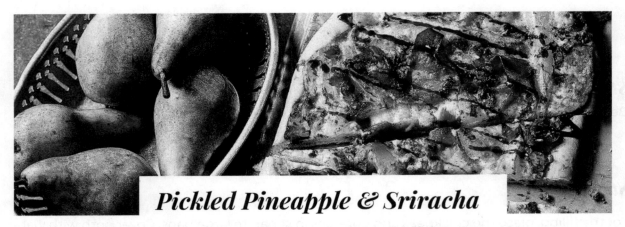

Pickled Pineapple & Sriracha
GRILLED CHEESE

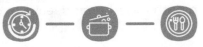

TIME
30

PREP TIME
10

SERVE
4

Directions:

Preheat oven to 400°F.

It starts from a cold, oven-safe pan over medium heat, cooking the bacon, 8 to 10 minutes, or crispy on both sides. Remove and set aside.

Season the chicken thigh with salt and pepper on both sides, then sear, skin-side down, in the bacon fat, 2 to 3 minutes. Turn chicken over, transfer pan to the oven, and roast for 15 minutes, or until cooked through. Set aside to cool slightly, then carve into bite-size pieces.

Lay the radicchio in one even layer on the largest plate you've got. Sprinkle over the malt vinegar, olive oil, and salt and pepper. (Sometimes, I do a pinch of sugar to offset the bitterness.)

Assemble the salad: In six color-blocked compartments over the radicchio, arrange the bacon, chicken, blue cheese, tomatoes, avocado, and egg, so the plate is bulging with FOOD. Season the tomatoes, avocado, and egg with salt and pepper, then garnish the entire plate with chives.

Ingredients:

- 3 to 4 slices bacon, cut in half
- 1 bone-in, skin-on chicken thigh
- Kosher salt and freshly ground black pepper, to taste
- 1/2 head radicchio, cut into quarters, so you're left with triangles (or however the heck you want to do it)
- 1 tablespoon malt vinegar
- 2 tablespoons extra-virgin olive oil
- 1-ounce blue cheese, chunked, at room temperature
- 1 handful cherry or Campari tomatoes, cut in half
- 1/2 avocado, thinly sliced
- 1 large organic egg, boiled for 7 to 8 minutes, peeled, then quartered
- 1 tablespoon chives, finely chopped

Roasted Seaweed Caesar Salad With

ANCHOVY CROUTONS

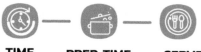

TIME
30

PREP TIME
15

SERVE
4

Directions:

Preheat oven to 350°F. Wash the lettuce leaves, spin or pat dry, then transfer to the refrigerator to keep cold and crisp until ready to dress.

Make the croutons: In a sheet pan or small baking dish, toss sourdough bread pieces with 1 tablespoon of the anchovy oil. Season with salt and pepper if desired (I prefer these croutons without seasoning because their bread-y sweetness balances the salty, punchy dressing). Bake for 10 to 15 minutes, or until crispy and lightly browned at the edges.

Meanwhile, make the dressing: In a small food processor, blitz the remaining tablespoon of anchovy oil, anchovies, garlic, egg yolk, rice vinegar, sesame oil, Worcestershire sauce, Parmesan cheese, and roasted seaweed snack until smooth and emulsified, scraping the sides in between pulses. It will be very thick; don't worry. Season lightly with salt (the anchovies and Parm are already pretty salty) and heavily with pepper (because it rules).

Transfer dressing into a large bowl. Take the cold romaine out of the fridge and toss it in the bowl

Ingredients:

- 1 romaine heart, separated into individual leaves
- 1 cup torn 1-inch pieces sourdough bread, crusts removed
- 6 anchovy fillets packed in olive oil (plus 2 tablespoons of the oil, divided)
- 1 fat garlic clove
- 1 large organic egg yolk
- 2 tablespoons rice vinegar
- 2 teaspoons sesame oil
- 1/2 teaspoon Worcestershire sauce
- 2 tablespoons finely grated Parmesan cheese, plus more for garnish
- 1 (5-gram) packet roasted seaweed snack, crushed with your hands
- Kosher salt
- Freshly ground black pepper

(I like to use my hands here to massage the dressing into each leave's nook and cranny). Add the croutons and toss gently one last time, tasting for seasoning. More salt? More pepper? Now's the time to adjust.

Transfer salad to a plate, piling the leaves high and scattering the croutons. Grate over a final dusting of Parmesan cheese and freshly ground black pepper. All salads wilt, but this one especially, so eat immediately.

CORNISH GAME HEN SOUP

With Garlic, Ginger & Fried Shallots

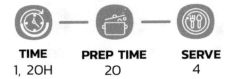

TIME
1, 20H

PREP TIME
20

SERVE
4

Direction

Place the rice in a sieve and run it under the tap for a few seconds to rinse off some of the excess starch. Transfer to a small bowl and cover with water. Let soak for 10 minutes.

Then, prepare the hen: Remove the pouch from inside the chicken's cavity. Add 4 or so garlic cloves into the cavity, and, using a spoon, add the rice as well.

Place stuffed chicken into a small pot or saucepan (it should be nice and snug). Sprinkle over the salt and pepper. Add remaining garlic cloves, ginger, and onion around the hen and fill the pot with water. (The hen doesn't need to be completely submerged; in fact, it shouldn't be, so the white meat can slowly steam in the covered pot while the dark meat braises and gets effortlessly tender in its garlicky, gingery hot bath.) Bring to a boil, cover, and reduce heat to low and cook for about 1 hour, spooning over some of the broth a couple of times during cooking.

Meanwhile, in a small saucepan, add the shallots and olive oil and bring to a gentle simmer, over low heat, and let cook, occasionally stirring, until shallots start to brown. This can take anywhere from 20 to 30 minutes, depending on your stove. Using a slotted spoon, remove the shallots and transfer to a paper towel to

Ingredients:

- 1/4 cup glutinous (sweet) rice or any other short-grain white rice
- 1 Cornish game hen (about 1 to 1 1/2 pounds)
- 8 garlic cloves
- 1 (2-inch) piece fresh ginger
- 1/4 small yellow onion
- 1 teaspoon kosher salt, plus more to taste
- 1/2 teaspoon ground white pepper, plus more to taste
- Water, as needed
- 1/4 cup thinly sliced shallots (about 1 small shallot)
- 1/4 cup olive oil
- 1 small bunch of fresh cilantro
- 1 bay leaf

drain. Save the oil; in fact, season it now with a little salt and white pepper. This will be your dipping sauce for the chicken later.

After an hour, the chicken should be cooked through and super tender. Season soup with additional salt and pepper, as needed, and garnish with fresh cilantro leaves and fried shallots. Eat straight out of its little pot with the shallot-y dipping sauce.

Pickled Radish
TACOS

TIME 40 — **PREP TIME** 20 — **SERVE** 4

Direction

Preheat a toaster oven or oven to 400°F. Place the majority of the radishes, their tops, the olive oil, the tomatillo, half the jalapeño in a bowl, season with salt and pepper, and toss. Remove the tomatillo and jalapeño, and place to one side of the roasting pan. Add the cumin and cinnamon to the bowl with the radishes and toss again. Remove the radishes and place them on the other side of the roasting pan. Bake until everything is softened, about 12– 15 minutes.

In the meantime, make the radish pickles: Cut the remaining three radishes into thin rounds and place in a small ramekin or bowl along with the onions, the other half of the jalapeño, and the smashed garlic. In a small sauté pan, bring the vinegar, three tablespoons of water, and a pinch of salt to a boil, then pour over the sliced radish mixture. (Note: If your radishes are on the larger side and the brine amount looks scant, you can easily double it.) Set aside to cool to room temperature.

When the roasting vegetables are soft, remove the tomatillo and jalapeño and place them in the container that came with your immersion blender (alternatively, you can use a mini food processor). Add the radish greens to the baking pan and replace them in the oven. Cook until wilted and remove. Taste and adjust salt and pepper. Place the remaining third of the garlic clove with the tomatillo and jalapeño, add the sprig of cilantro, the teaspoon of lime juice, and the remaining water, and blend with the hand blender, to make a smooth salsa. Season to taste with salt and pepper. If the salsa is looking thin and you'd like to bulk it up, you can add some of the wilted radish tops to the blender and blend till smooth.

Ingredients:

- 1 bunch radishes with tops intact, washed (reserve the tops and the 3 smallest radishes for later; quarter the rest)
- 2 tablespoons olive oil
- one 2-inch tomatillo, husk removed, cut in half
- 1 small jalapeño, stem removed, cut lengthwise (or to taste: jalapeños vary greatly on the Scoville scale, so keep that in mind when using)
- Salt and black pepper to taste
- 1 large pinch cumin
- 1 small pinch of cinnamon
- one 1/3-inch slice medium onion
- 1 clove garlic (smash 2/3, set aside remaining 1/3)
- 2 tablespoons white vinegar or cider vinegar (or more as needed)
- 5 tablespoons water
- 1 sprig cilantro
- 1 teaspoon lime juice
- To serve: 4 small corn tortillas, 1/4 cup queso fresco, crumbled, a wedge of lime (optional—there should be enough acidity from the pickles and salsa)

Reheat the tortillas in a dry, hot saute pan or on top of the toaster oven, one by one. Make the tacos with the roasted radishes and tops, garnished with a little salsa, pickles, and queso fresco. (Serve with wedges of lime if desired.)

CHAPTER 13
Late-Night Meal

THE "BIG SALAD"

"After a long day, the easiest and most satisfying meal to make is a Seinfeld-style' big salad'! I love crunchy lettuce, so I make sure to have romaine hearts or iceberg lettuce in the refrigerator at all times. Cucumber, tomato, and red onion are always included, but the key ingredients to bring this gem of a salad together are artichoke hearts, pepperoncini peppers, and hard salami. I top it off with a homemade dressing made out of red wine vinegar, olive oil, dried oregano, salt, and pepper. The best part of this meal is that I put all ingredients into a huge pot, mix it up and eat it right out of the pot, no other plating necessary!

THE GLUTINOUS RAGING WAF-FLE SANDWICH

"Use leftover waffles or frozen waffles from your freezer to make a sandwich. Use a skillet to make a hot ham, bacon & American cheese waffle sandwich. Add lettuce, tomato, and mustard, honey aioli sauce. If you want to get fun with it, you can also add crushed up potato chips drenched in hot sauce to your sandwich to offer a satisfying crunch."

THE KITCHEN SINK FRIED RICE

"I almost always have leftover takeout rice, eggs, and some random combination of Asian condiments in my refrigerator, so when I need a quick late-nick snack, I'm looking for some way to throw all those ingredients in a bowl. I scramble eggs into the rice and cook slowly while I get all my other toppings together. My favorite combination is gochujang, toasted sesame seeds or togarashi, green onions, and cilantro. If I have any crunchy vegetables, I'll toss that in some rice vinegar and put it on top to feel better about my life choices!

THE GLUTINOUS RAGING WAFFLE SANDWICH

"Use leftover waffles or frozen waffles from your freezer to make a sandwich. Use a skillet to make a hot ham, bacon & American cheese waffle sandwich. Add lettuce, tomato, and mustard, honey aioli sauce. If you want to get fun with it, you can also add crushed up potato chips drenched in hot sauce to your sandwich to offer a satisfying crunch."

CHAPTER 14
Salad

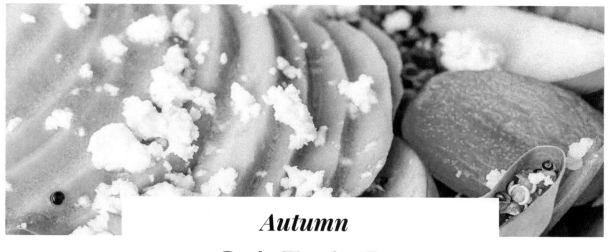

Autumn

SALAD

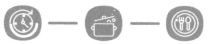

TIME	PREP TIME	SERVE
25	15	4

The flavor contrasts in this salad are lovely, and I've kept the pear to a the quantity that won't add too many carbs.

Directions:

Melt the butter in a small, heavy skillet over medium heat. Add the walnuts, and let they toast in the butter, occasionally stirring, for about 5 minutes.

While the walnuts are toasting-and make sure you keep an eye on them and don't burn them-wash and dry your greens, and put them in a salad bowl with the onion.

Toss with the oil first, then combine the vinegar, lemon juice, mustard, salt, and pepper, and add that to the salad bowl. Toss until everything is well covered.

Top the salad with the pear, the warm toasted walnuts, and the crumbled blue cheese; serve.

Notes

4 generous servings, each with 13 grams of carbohydrates and 6 grams of fiber, for a total of 7 grams of usable carbs and 10 grams of protein.

Ingredients:

- 2 tablespoons butter
- 1/2 cup chopped walnuts
- 10 cups loosely packed assorted greens (romaine, red leaf lettuce, and fresh spinach)
- 1/4 sweet red onion, thinly sliced
- 1/4 cup olive oil
- 2 teaspoons wine vinegar
- 2 teaspoons lemon juice
- 1/4 teaspoon spicy brown or Dijon mustard
- 1/8 teaspoon salt
- 1/8 teaspoon pepper
- 1/2 ripe pear, chopped
- 1/3 cup crumbled blue cheese

CHAPTER 15
Homemade Beef

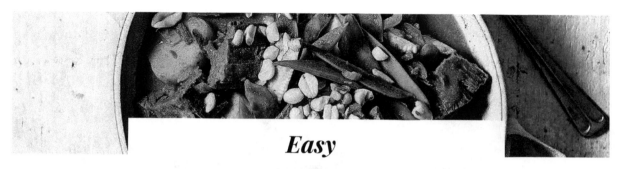

Easy

BEEF STEW

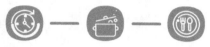

TIME	PREP TIME	SERVE
1h30m	20	1

Beef stew meat is often made from the ends of different cuts of beef. If your beef is not tender after 60 minutes, cover and allow to simmer an additional 15-20 minutes or until tender..

Directions:

Combine flour, garlic powder, and salt & pepper. Toss beef in flour mixture. Heat olive oil in a large Dutch oven or pot. Cook the beef and onions until browned. Add beef broth and red wine while scraping up any brown bits in the pan. Stir in all remaining ingredients except for peas, cornstarch, and water. Reduce heat to medium-low, cover, and simmer 1 hour or until beef is tender (up to 90 minutes). Mix equal parts of cornstarch and water to create a slurry. Slowly add the slurry to the boiling stew to reach the desired consistency (you may not need all of the slurries). Stir in peas and simmer 5-10 minutes before serving. Season with salt & pepper to taste.

Ingredients:

- 2 pounds stewing beef trimmed and cubed
- 3 tablespoons flour
- ½ teaspoon garlic powder
- ½ teaspoon salt
- ½ teaspoon black pepper
- 3 tablespoons olive oil
- 1 onion chopped
- 6 cups beef broth
- ½ cup red wine optional
- 1 pound potatoes peeled and cubed
- 4 carrots cut into 1-inch pieces
- 4 stalks celery cut into 1-inch pieces
- 3 tablespoons tomato paste
- 1 teaspoon dried rosemary or 1 sprig fresh
- 2 tablespoons cornstarch
- 2 tablespoons water
- ¾ cup peas

Notes

Calories: 444, Carbohydrates: 22g, Protein: 25g, Fat: 28g, Saturated Fat: 9g, Cholesterol: 80mg, Sodium: 383mg, Potassium: 1105mg, Fiber: 4g, Sugar: 4g, Vitamin A: 5755IU, Vitamin C: 27.1mg, Calcium: 73mg, Iron: 5.5mg

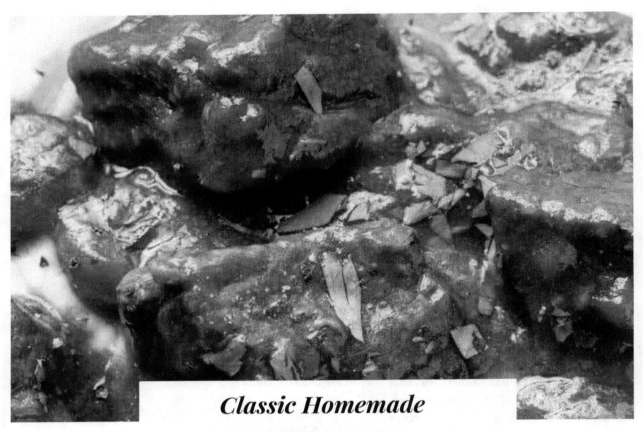

Classic Homemade

BEEF

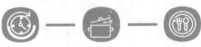

TIME	PREP TIME	SERVE
2h 25m	20	4

Ingredients:

- 1/4 cup all-purpose flour
- 1/4 teaspoon black pepper
- 2 lb. chuck pot roast, trimmed and cut into 3/4" pieces
- 3 tablespoons vegetable oil
- 3 cups vegetable juice (such as V8)
- 3 cups beef broth

- 2 medium onions, cut into thin wedges
- 1 cup thinly sliced celery
- 2 tablespoons Worcestershire sauce
- 1 teaspoon dried thyme
- 1 bay leaf
- 4 red potatoes, cut into 1-inch cubes
- 4 carrots, peeled and cut into 1/4-inch slices on a bias
- 1 1/2 cups frozen peas

Directions:

Place the flour and the pepper in a large resealable plastic bag. Add the beef, seal the bag, and shake until all the pieces are coated with the flour mixture.

In a 5 to 6 quart Dutch oven or heavy pot, heat half of the vegetable oil over medium-high heat. Add half of the beef and cook until browned on all sides. Remove the beef to a plate, add more oil, and cook the remaining beef.

When the beef is browned, return all of the beef to the pot. Stir in the vegetable juice, beef broth, onion, celery, Worcestershire sauce, thyme, and bay leaf. Bring to a boil, then reduce the heat and cover and cook for 1 hour.

Stir the potatoes and carrots into the stew. Return to a boil, reduce the heat and cover, and cook for an additional 30 to 40 minutes, or until the vegetables are tender.

Stir in the peas and cook until heated through. Remove the bay leaf and serve.

Recipe Notes:

Nutrition information is provided as an estimate only. Various brands and products can change the counts. Any nutritional information should only be used as a general guideline.

Nutrition:

Serving Size: 1/8 of recipe Calories: 337 Sugar: 27 g Sodium: 658 mg Fat: 9 g Saturated Fat: 2 g Unsaturated Fat: 4 g Trans Fat: 0 g Carbohydrates: 29 g Fiber: 5 g Protein: 27 g Cholesterol: 65 mg

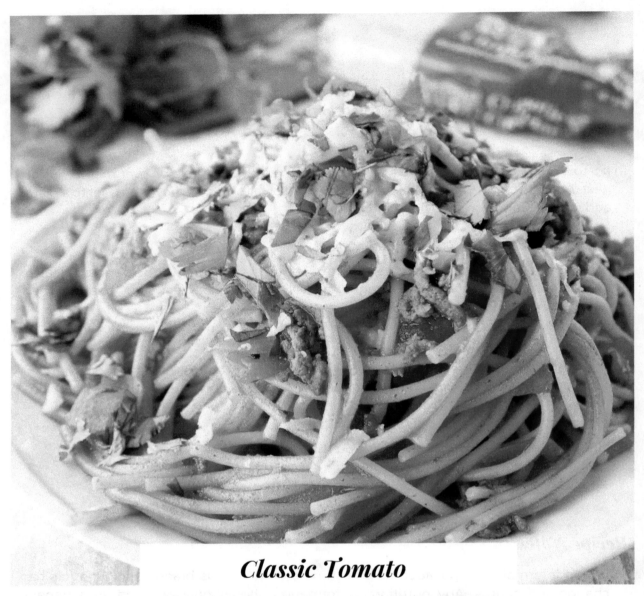

Classic Tomato

SPAGHETTI

Ingredients:

- 1 bunch of fresh basil
- 1 medium onion
- 2 cloves of garlic

- 1 kg ripe tomatoes, or 2 x 400g tins of quality chopped tomatoes olive oil
- 1 tablespoon red wine or balsamic vinegar
- 480 g dried wholewheat spaghetti
- 15 g Parmesan cheese

Directions:

Pick the basil leaves onto a chopping board (reserving a few babies leaves to garnish), then roughly chop the remaining leaves and finely chop the stalks.

Peel and finely slice the onion and garlic. If using fresh, cut the tomatoes in half, then roughly chop them or carefully open tomatoes' tins.

Put a saucepan on medium heat and add 1 tablespoon of olive oil and the onion, then cook for around 7 minutes, or until soft and lightly golden.

Stir in the garlic and basil stalks for a few minutes, then add the fresh or tinned tomatoes and the vinegar.

Season with a tiny pinch of salt and pepper, then continue cooking for around 15 minutes, stirring occasionally.

Stir in the chopped basil leaves, then reduce to low and leave to tick away. Meanwhile...

Carefully fill large pot three-quarters of the way up with boiling water, add a tiny pinch of salt and bring back to the boil.

Add the spaghetti and cook according to packet instructions – you want to cook your pasta until it is al dente. This translates as 'to the tooth' and means that it should be soft enough to eat but still have a bit of a bite and firmness. Use the timings on the packet instructions as a guide, but try some just before the time is up to make sure it's perfectly cooked.

Once the pasta is done, scoop out and reserve a cup of the cooking water, keep it to one side, drain in a colander over the sink, and tip the spaghetti back into the pot.

Stir the spaghetti into the sauce, adding a splash of the pasta water to loosen, if needed.

Serve with the reserved basil leaves sprinkled over the top and used a Microplane to grate the Parmesan cheese, then sprinkle over finely.

CHAPTER 16
Drink

Hot
APPLE CIDER

Directions:

Pour the apple cider and maple syrup into a large stainless steel saucepan.

Place the cinnamon sticks, cloves, allspice berries, orange peel, and lemon peel in the center of a washed square of cheesecloth; fold up the cheesecloth's sides to enclose the bundle, then tie it up with a length of kitchen string. Drop the spice bundle into the cider mixture.

Place the saucepan over moderate heat for 5 to 10 minutes, or until the cider is very hot but not boiling. Remove the cider from the heat. Discard the spice bundle. Ladle the cider into big cups or mugs, adding a fresh cinnamon stick to each serving if desired.

Ingredients:

- 6 cups apple cider
- ¼ cup real maple syrup
- 2 cinnamon sticks
- 6 whole cloves
- 6 whole allspice berries
- 1 orange peel, cut into strips
- 1 lemon peel, cut into strips

TIME	PREP TIME	SERVE
15	10	6

Rudolph
TINI

Ingredients:

- 2 fluid ounces vodka
- 1 fluid ounce hazelnut liqueur, such as Frangelico
- 1 fluid ounce coconut-flavored rum
- 1 fluid ounce half-and-half cream
- 2 (4 inches) cinnamon sticks
- 1 maraschino cherry

Directions:

Pour the vodka, hazelnut liqueur, rum, and half-and-half into a cocktail shaker over ice. Cover, and shake until the outside of the shaker has frosted. Strain into a chilled martini glass; garnish with the cinnamon sticks to look like antlers and the cherry on the rim to look like a nose.

TIME	PREP TIME	SERVE
5	5	1

Candy Cane
COCOA

Directions:

In a saucepan, heat milk until hot but not boiling. Whisk in the chocolate and the crushed peppermint candies until melted and smooth. Pour hot cocoa into four mugs, and garnish with whipped cream. Serve each with a candy cane stirring stick.

Per Serving: 486 calories; protein 10g; carbohydrates 80.2g; fat 14.9g; cholesterol 30.9mg; sodium 140.8mg.

Ingredients:

- 4 cups of milk
- 3 (1 ounce) squares semisweet chocolate, chopped
- 4 peppermint candy canes, crushed
- 1 cup whipped cream
- 4 small peppermint candy canes

TIME	PREP TIME	SERVE
5	15	4

Slow Cooker
CHAI

Ingredients:

- 2 fluid ounces vodka
- 1 fluid ounce hazelnut liqueur, such as Frangelico
- 1 fluid ounce coconut-flavored rum
- 1 fluid ounce half-and-half cream
- 2 (4 inches) cinnamon sticks
- 1 maraschino cherry

Directions:

Pour water into the crock of a slow cooker. Stir in the ginger, cardamom pods, cloves, cinnamon sticks, and peppercorns. Turn to High; simmer for 8 hours.

Steep tea bags in the hot spiced water for 5 minutes. Strain tea into a clean container. Stir in sweetened condensed milk; serve hot.

TIME	PREP TIME	SERVE
8H 25m	5	16

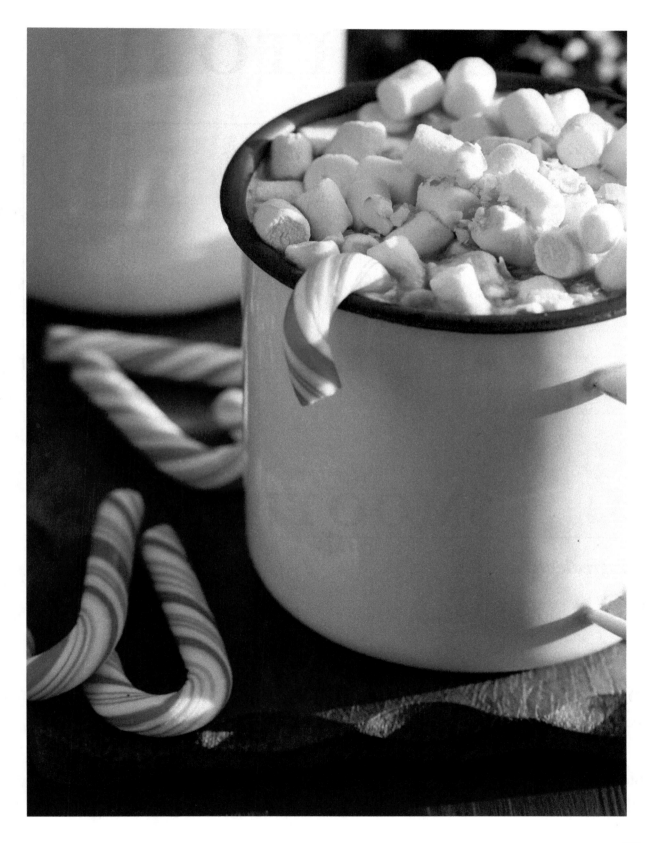

COQUITO II

Directions:

In a medium bowl, whisk egg yolks until smooth. Whisk in cinnamon and vanilla. Stir in coconut milk, cream of coconut sweetened condensed milk evaporated milk and rum. Taste and adjust cinnamon and vanilla if desired. Blend well and strain through a fine sieve or cheesecloth. Pour into clean bottles. Serve chilled.

Per Serving: Per Serving: 503 calories; protein 10.6g; carbohydrates 39.2g; fat 18.6g; cholesterol 42.6mg; sodium 168.2mg.

Ingredients:

- 6 egg yolks
- ½ teaspoon ground cinnamon
- 4 tablespoons vanilla extract
- 1 (14 ounces) can sweeten condensed milk
- 5 (12 fluid ounce) cans of evaporated milk
- 1 (10 ounces) can unsweetened coconut milk
- 1 (14 ounces) can sweeten cream of coconut
- 4 ¼ cups light rum

TIME	PREP TIME	SERVE
35	35	15

Starter
SMOOTHIE

Ingredients:

- 2 fluid ounces vodka
- 1 fluid ounce hazelnut liqueur, such as Frangelico
- 1 fluid ounce coconut-flavored rum
- 1 fluid ounce half-and-half cream
- 2 (4 inches) cinnamon sticks
- 1 maraschino cherry

Directions:

Pour water into the crock of a slow cooker. Stir in the ginger, cardamom pods, cloves, cinnamon sticks, and peppercorns. Turn to High; simmer for 8 hours.

Steep tea bags in the hot spiced water for 5 minutes. Strain tea into a clean container. Stir in sweetened

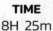

TIME	PREP TIME	SERVE
8H 25m	5	16

condensed milk; serve hot.

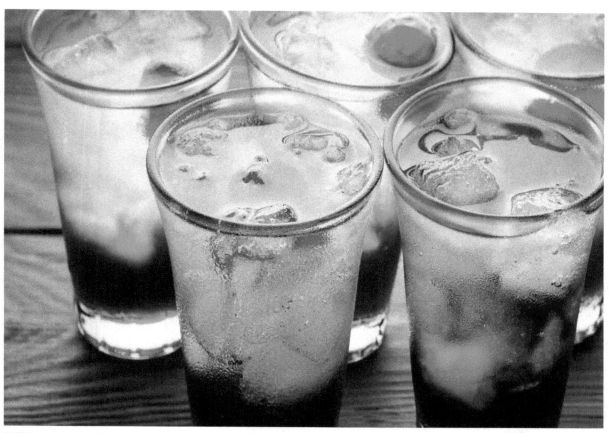

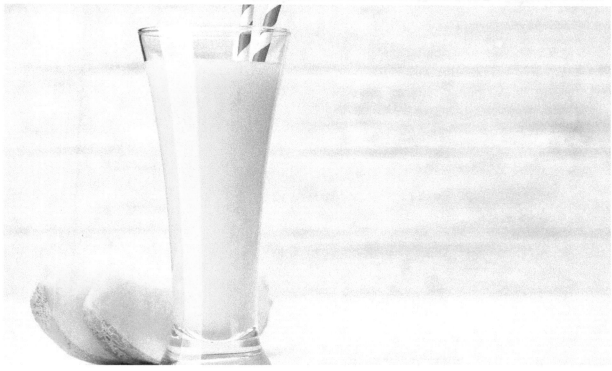

CHAPTER 17
Drink

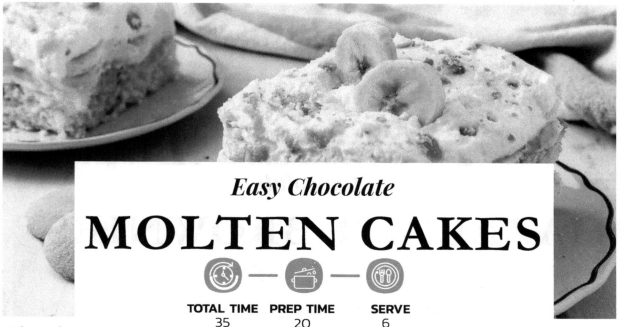

Easy Chocolate
MOLTEN CAKES

TOTAL TIME	PREP TIME	SERVE
35	20	6

Directions:

Step 1

Heat oven to 200C/180C fan/gas 6. Butter 6 dariole molds or basins well and place on a baking tray.

Step 2

Put 100g butter and 100g chopped dark chocolate in a heatproof bowl and set over a pan of hot water (or put in the microwave and melt in 30-second bursts on a low setting) and stir until smooth. Set aside to cool slightly for 15 mins.

Step 3

Using an electric hand whisk, mix in 150g light brown soft sugar, then 3 large eggs, one at a time, followed by ½ tsp vanilla extract and finally 50g plain flour. Divide the mixture among the darioles or basins.

Step 4

You can now either put the mixture in the fridge or freezer until you're ready to bake them. Can be cooked straight from frozen for 16 mins, or bake

Ingredients:

- 100g butter, plus extra to grease
- 100g dark chocolate, chopped
- 150g light brown soft sugar
- 3 large eggs
- ½ tsp vanilla extract
- 50g plain flour

Step 5

Carefully run a knife around each pudding edge, then turn out onto serving plates and serve with single cream.

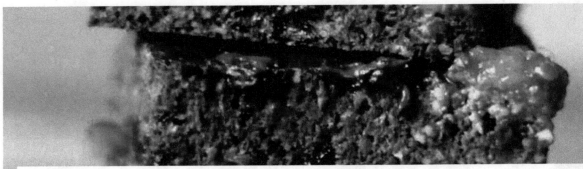

Salted Chocolate &

HAZELNUT BROWNIES

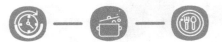

TOTAL TIME	PREP TIME	SERVE
35	20	6

Directions:

Step 1

Heat oven to 180C/160C fan/ gas 4. Butter and line the base and sides of a 20cm square tin. Put the butter, chocolate and chocolate spread in a heatproof bowl and melt over a pan of lightly simmering water. Once melted, stir and set aside to cool a little.

Step 2

In another bowl, use an electric whisk to beat the eggs and sugar together for 5 mins until light and fluffy. Pour in the chocolate mixture and whisk briefly to combine. Sift in the flour and gently fold through the mixture, then add most of the pecans. Scrape the mixture into the tin and spread out with a spatula. Scatter over the last of the pecans and a good sprinkling of sea salt.

Step 3

Bake for 30-35 mins until set but a little gooey in the middle. Cool, then cut into squares and serve with ice cream and caramel sauce.

Ingredients:

- 100g slightly salted butter, cut into small pieces, plus extra for the tin
- 200g 70% dark chocolate, broken into chunks
- 150g chocolate and hazelnut spread
- 3 eggs, beaten
- 200g golden caster sugar
- 150g plain flour
- 100g toasted pecan nuts, roughly chopped
- ice cream and caramel sauce, to serve
- single cream, to serve

PEACH MELBA PIE

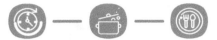

TOTAL TIME
35

PREP TIME
20

SERVE
6

Directions:

Step 1

Combine both flours, the butter, and a pinch of salt in the bowl of a food processor and blitz to a fine crumb. Add cold water 1 tbsp at a time (4-5 tbsp), pulsing until the mix starts to cling together. Tip out and knead with your hands (add more water if required) to make

Step 2

Remove a disc of pastry from the fridge, unwrap and, on a generously floured surface, roll it out to a large circle, wider than the pie dish. Transfer to a floured baking sheet and chill for about 10 mins. Repeat with the remaining disc.

Step 3

Heat the oven to 180C/160C fan/gas 4. Stone and quarter the peaches. Cut each in two, and toss in a bowl with the lemon juice, cornflour, vanilla extract, sugar, honey, and raspberries. Add the butter in small pieces.

Step 4

Using a floured rolling pin, drape one of the pastry sheets across a 24cm pie dish. Let it sink in and, holding the edges, lift and tuck into the corners. Prick the pastry all over and fill with the peach mixture.

Step 5

Drape the second pastry sheet over the filling. Press together the top and bottom crusts, crimping with your fingers to seal, and trim off any excess. Cut three 8cm slits across the top crust, brush with the beaten egg and sprinkle over the demerara sugar. Bake for 55 mins to 1 hr until the crust is deeply golden and the filling is bubbling out. Cool for about 10 mins before serving with cream or vanilla ice cream.

Ingredients:

- 175g self-raising flour, plus extra for dusting
- 175g white spelled flour
- 160g unsalted butter, chilled and cubed
- For the filling
- 4 ripe peaches
- ½ lemon, juiced
- 1 tbsp cornflour
- 1 tsp vanilla extract
- 3 tbsp light muscovado sugar
- 1 tbsp runny blossom honey
- 200g raspberries
- 10g chilled butter
- 1 egg, beaten
- 2 tbsp demerara sugar
- vanilla ice cream or

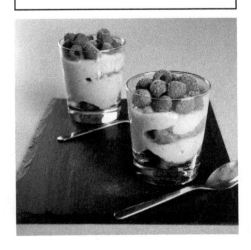

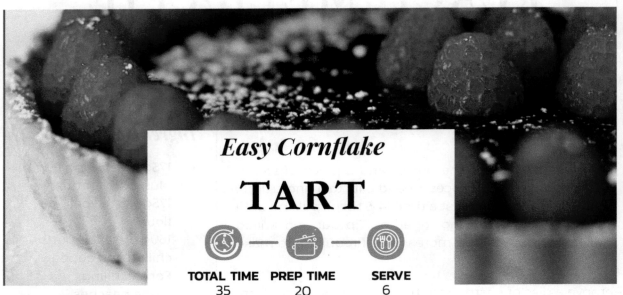

Easy Cornflake
TART

TOTAL TIME 35 — **PREP TIME** 20 — **SERVE** 6

Directions:

Step 1

Heat the oven to 180C/160C fan/gas 4. Unroll the pastry and briefly roll out on a lightly floured work surface until it's large enough to fit a 23cm loose-bottomed tart tin. Use the rolling pin to lift the pastry over the tin, then press into the corners and sides, so the excess pastry hangs over the rim. Trim this away, leaving just a small amount of excess hanging over the rim.

Step 2

Line the pastry with baking parchment and fill with baking beans or uncooked rice. Bake for 15 mins. Remove the parchment and beans, then bake for another 5-10 mins until just golden. Remove from the oven and trim any excess pastry from the edges using a serrated knife.

Step 3

Heat the butter, syrup, and sugar in a small pan with a pinch of salt, frequently stirring, until melted and smooth. Fold in the cornflakes to coat in the butter mixture.

Step 4

Spoon the jam into the cooked pastry base, then level

Ingredients:

- 320g ready-rolled shortcrust pastry
- plain flour, to dust
- 50g butter
- 125g golden syrup
- 25g light brown soft sugar
- 100g cornflakes
- 125g strawberry or raspberry jam custard, to serve

the surface. Tip the cornflake mixture over the jam and gently press down until all of the jam is covered with a mixture layer. Return the tart to the oven and bake for another 5 mins until the cornflakes are golden and toasted. Leave to cool until just warm before slicing and serving with custard.

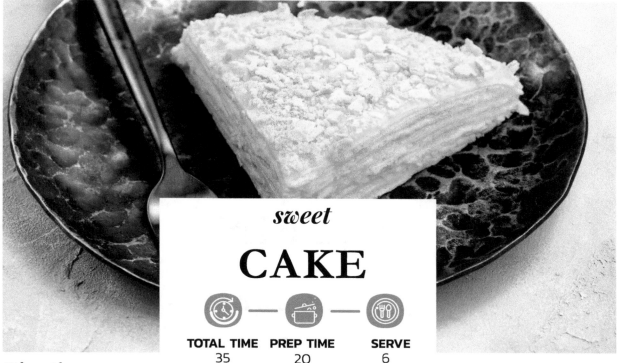

sweet

CAKE

TOTAL TIME	PREP TIME	SERVE
35	20	6

Directions:

Step 1

Preheat oven to 425°. Line a baking sheet with parchment paper.

Step 2

Combine the first 4 ingredients in a large bowl. Cut butter into flour mixture with a pastry blender or fork until mixture resembles fine crumbs.

Step 3

Whisk together cream and egg; add to dry ingredients, stirring just until the dough comes together. (Dough will be sticky.) Turn dough out onto a lightly floured surface; knead with floured hands 4 or 5 times. Pat to 1 1/2-inch thickness. Cut into 6 rounds with a 2 1/2-inch round cutter, and place 2 inches apart on a prepared baking sheet.

Ingredients:

- 2 cups all-purpose flour
- ¼ cup of sugar
- 1 tablespoon baking powder
- ½ teaspoon salt
- ½ cup butter, cut into pieces
- ½ cup cream or whole milk
- 1 large egg, lightly beaten

Step 4

Bake 12 to 15 minutes or until golden. Cool completely.

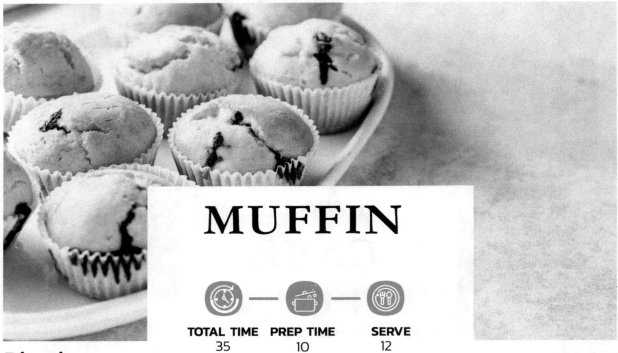

MUFFIN

TOTAL TIME	PREP TIME	SERVE
35	10	12

Directions:

Step 1

Preheat oven to 400 degrees F (205 degrees C).

Step 2

Stir together the flour, baking powder, salt, and sugar in a large bowl. Make a well in the center. In a small bowl or 2 cup measuring cup, beat egg with a fork. Stir in milk and oil. Pour all at once into the well in the flour mixture. Mix quickly and lightly with a fork until moistened, but do not beat. The batter will be lumpy. Pour the batter into paper-lined muffin pan cups.

Ingredients:

- 2 cups all-purpose flour
- 3 teaspoons baking powder
- ½ teaspoon salt
- ¾ cup white sugar
- 1 egg
- 1 cup milk
- ¼ cup of vegetable oil
- beaten

Step 3

Variations: Blueberry Muffins: Add 1 cup fresh blueberries. Raisin Muffins: Add 1 cup finely chopped raisins. Date Muffins: Add 1 cup finely chopped dates. Cheese Muffins: Fold in 1 cup grated sharp yellow cheese. Bacon Muffins: Fold 1/4 cup crisp cooked bacon, broken into bits. **Bake for 25 minutes, or until golden.**

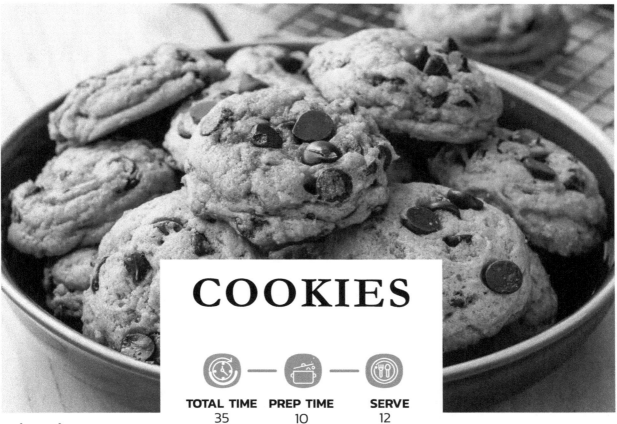

COOKIES

TOTAL TIME 35 — **PREP TIME** 10 — **SERVE** 12

Directions:

Step 1

Heat oven to 350°F. In a large bowl, whisk together heavy cream and eggs. Stir in bacon, cheese, and thyme.

Step 2

Pour egg mixture into pie crust and bake 40 to 50 minutes or until knife inserted in center comes out clean.

Step 3

Let cool 5 to 10 minutes and garnish with parsley before serving.

Ingredients:

- 1 refrigerated pie crust (or homemade pie dough)
- 6 large eggs
- 3/4 c. heavy cream
- 6 slices bacon, cooked and crumbled
- 1 c. shredded Gruyère cheese
- 1 tsp. thyme leaves
- Kosher salt
- Pinch cayenne
- Freshly ground black pepper
- 2 tbsp. freshly chopped parsley

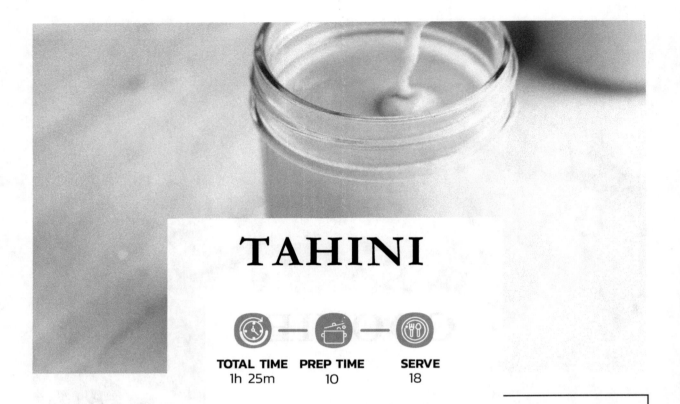

TAHINI

TOTAL TIME
1h 25m

PREP TIME
10

SERVE
18

Directions:

Preheat oven to 350° and line 2 two baking sheets with parchment. In a medium bowl, whisk together flour, baking powder, baking soda, and salt.

In a large bowl, using a hand mixer, beat butter and sugars together until combined. Add eggs, one at a time beating well after each egg, then add vanilla and tahini and beat until creamy. Add dry ingredients and beat until just combined.

Roll about 2 tablespoons of dough into a ball, then roll in sesame seeds and place on prepared baking sheets 2" apart. The dough will be soft but shouldn't stick to your hands.

Bake until the edges are lightly golden and just set, but middles are still soft, 13 to 14 minutes.

Let cool on baking sheet for 5 minutes, then move to a cooling rack to cool completely.

Ingredients:

- 2 1/4 c. all-purpose flour
- 1 tsp. baking powder
- 1/2 tsp. baking soda
- 1/2 tsp. kosher salt
- 1/2 c. (1 stick) butter softened
- 3/4 c. packed brown sugar
- 1/2 c. granulated sugar
- 2 large eggs
- 1 tsp. pure vanilla extract
- 3/4 c. tahini
- 1/2 c. sesame seeds

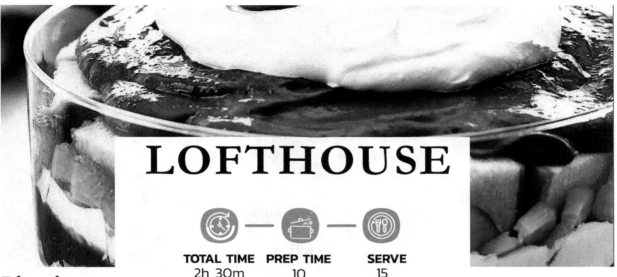

LOFTHOUSE

TOTAL TIME
2h 30m

PREP TIME
10

SERVE
15

Directions:

In a large bowl, whisk together flour, cornstarch, baking powder, and salt. In another large bowl, using a hand mixer, beat butter, cream cheese, and sugar together until light and fluffy. Add egg and extracts and beat until well combined. Add dry ingredients and beat until just combined. Transfer dough to plastic wrap and smooth into a disc. The dough will still be soft and sticky at this point. Refrigerate until well chilled, at least 1 hour. Preheat oven to 350° and line 2 large baking sheets with parchment. Lightly flour surface and place dough on the counter. Dust top of the dough with flour as well. Roll dough out to ½" thick. Use a 3" round cookie cutter to cut cookies and place on prepared baking sheets 2" apart. Gather scraps and re-roll to cut out more cookies. Bake until edges are just set, but centers are still slightly underdone, 10 to 12 minutes. Cookies shouldn't gain many colors on top. Let cool completely on baking sheets. Meanwhile, make the frosting: In a large bowl using a hand mixer, beat butter until completely smooth and creamy, 2 minutes. Add powdered sugar and beat again until light and fluffy, about 3 minutes more. Add heavy cream, vanilla, and a pinch of salt and beat until combined. Add desired food coloring and beat again to combine. Use an offset spatula to frost the tops of cooled cookies with a thick amount of frosting, then top with sprinkles.

Ingredients:

- For Cookies:
- 2 1/4 c. all-purpose flour, plus more for surface
- 1/4 c. cornstarch
- 1 tsp. baking powder
- 1 tsp. kosher salt
- 1/2 c. (1 stick) butter softened
- 4 oz. cream cheese softened
- 1 c. granulated sugar
- 1 large egg
- 1 tsp. pure vanilla extract
- 1/2 tsp. almond extract
- For Buttercream:
- 3/4 c. (1 1/2 sticks) butter softened
- 2 3/4 c. powdered sugar
- 1 tbsp. heavy cream
- 1 tsp. pure vanilla extract
- Pinch of kosher salt
- Food coloring
- Sprinkles, for decorating

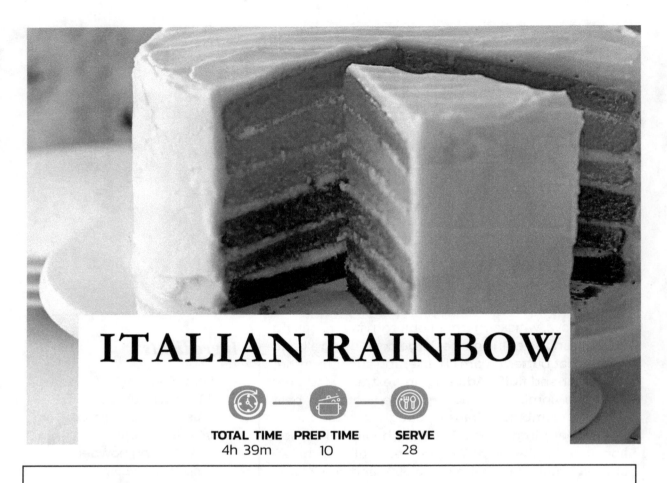

ITALIAN RAINBOW

TOTAL TIME
4h 39m

PREP TIME
10

SERVE
28

Ingredients:

- Cooking spray
- 7 oz. almond paste, broken into pieces
- 1 1/4 c. (2 1/2 sticks) butter softened
- 1 c. granulated sugar, divided
- 4 large eggs, separated
- 1 tsp. almond extract
- 2 3/4 c. all-purpose flour

- 1/2 tsp. kosher salt
- Red food coloring
- Green food coloring
- 1/3 c. apricot preserves, warmed
- 1/3 c. raspberry preserves, warmed
- 1 1/4 c. semisweet chocolate chips, divided

Directions:

Preheat oven to 350°. Grease three 9"-x-13" pans with cooking spray and line with parchment paper, leaving a 2" hangover on each side. In a large bowl using a hand mixer, beat almond paste and ¾ cup sugar together until light almond paste is broken into smaller pieces and looks crumbly. Add butter and beat until light and fluffy. Add egg yolks and almond extract and beat until incorporated. Add flour and salt and beat until just combined.

In another large bowl, beat egg whites until foamy, then slowly add in remaining ¼ cup sugar while beating and continue beating until stiff peaks. Add about ⅓ of the egg whites to the batter and gently fold in until combined, then add the rest of the egg whites and continue gently folding until fully combined.

Divide batter evenly into 3 separate bowls. Dye one bowl of batter red and another bowling green, leaving the third one plain. Add batters to prepared pans and use an offset spatula to spread into an even layer.

Bake until no longer shiny and feel just slightly soft when pressed with a finger, 12 minutes. The cakes should be starting to peel from the edges, and barely any color will be gained. Let cool 10 minutes in the pan, then use the parchment to lift out and place on cooling racks. Let cool completely.

To assemble the cakes, place parchment paper over the green layer, then invert layer onto aboard. Peel off the top piece of parchment paper. Spread warmed apricot preserves over green layer.

Invert the white layer onto another board and peel off the parchment paper. Gently slide it on top of the green layer. Spread warmed raspberry preserves over white layer. Finally, invert the red layer onto another board, peel off parchment, and gently slide on the white layer. Place a piece of parchment paper on top of the red layer, then place a baking pan on top of the parchment.

Weigh down the pan with cans and refrigerate for at least 2 hours or up to overnight.

When ready to coat in chocolate, remove it from the refrigerator while you temper your chocolate. To temper, your chocolate, place ¾ cup chocolate chips into a microwave-safe bowl. Microwave in 30-second intervals, stirring after each one until chocolate is smooth and reaches between 113° and 118°. Microwave in 5 to 10 seconds bursts as needed to hit your desired temperature. Add remaining ½ cup of chocolate chips a little at a time, stirring until completely melted between additions. Keep stirring until your chocolate reaches 88° or 89°. You can add a little more chocolate as needed to help cool your chocolate down, making sure the new chips melt completely before adding any more.

Add about half of your tempered chocolate on top of the red layer, and working quickly, so it doesn't set, use an offset spatula to spread into an even layer. Refrigerate until chocolate is completely set, 30 minutes.

If your chocolate hardened while the first layer was chilling, microwave in 10-second bursts until smooth and chocolate reach 89° again. Once the chocolate is set, invert onto another board and spread the remaining chocolate over the green layer. Refrigerate until chocolate is set or until ready to serve, 30 more minutes.

Using a large knife, trim edges of cakes to get clean sides, cut into 28 pieces.

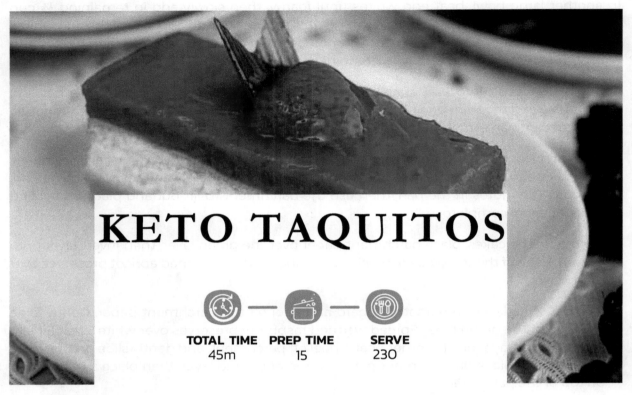

KETO TAQUITOS

TOTAL TIME
45m

PREP TIME
15

SERVE
230

Directions:

Preheat oven to 375° and line two baking sheets with parchment paper. In a medium skillet over medium heat, heat oil. Add onion and cook until slightly soft, 3 minutes. Add garlic and spices and cook until fragrant, 1 to 2 minutes more. Add chicken and enchilada sauce, then bring mixture to a simmer. Stir in cilantro, season with salt, and remove from heat.

Make taquito shells: In a medium bowl, mix cheeses. Divide mixture into twelve 3 ½" piles on a prepared baking sheet. Bake until cheese is melty and slightly golden around the edges, about 10 minutes. Let cool 2 to 4 minutes, then peel shells off parchment. Add a small pile of chicken to each and roll tightly. Repeat until all taquitos are made.

Garnish with cilantro and serve with sour cream for dipping.

Ingredients:

- 2 tbsp. extra-virgin olive oil
- 1/2 onion, finely chopped
- 4 cloves garlic, minced
- 1 tsp. ground cumin
- 1 tsp. chili powder
- 2 c. shredded chicken
- 2/3 c. red enchilada sauce
- 4 tbsp. freshly chopped cilantro, plus more for garnish
- Kosher salt
- 2 c. shredded cheddar
- 2 c. shredded Monterey jack
- Sour cream, for serving (optional)

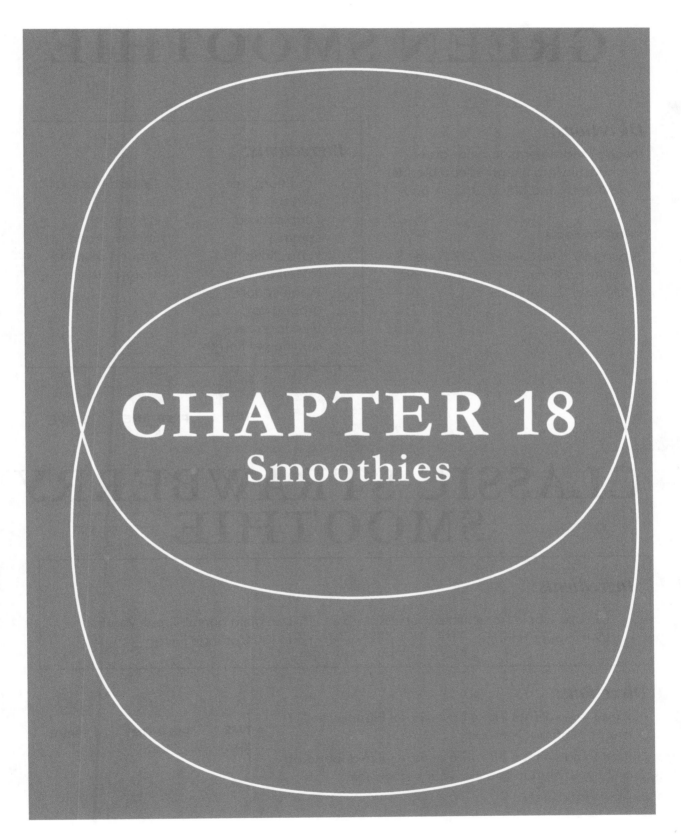

CHAPTER 18
Smoothies

GREEN SMOOTHIE

Directions:

Place all ingredients for your green smoothie into a high-speed blender or Vitamix and blend until smooth.

Nutrition Facts

Serving Size: 1/2 Calories: 327 Sugar: 34 Sodium: 135 Fat: 14 Carbohydrates: 53 Fiber: 12 Protein: 5

Ingredients:

- 1 medium frozen avocado
- 1 cup packed spinach
- 1 cup sliced frozen banana
- 1 tablespoon ground flax
- 1/4 cup frozen cauliflower florets
- 3 pitted Medjool dates
- 1.25 cups unsweetened almond milk (or more, to taste)

TIME	PREP TIME	SERVE
5	5	2

CLASSIC STRAWBERRY SMOOTHIE

Ingredients:

- 1.5 cups whole frozen strawberries
- 1/2 medium banana
- 1/2 cup plain nonfat Greek yogurt
- 1 cup 100% orange juice

Directions:

Place all ingredients into a high-speed blender and mix on high until smooth.

Option to add a little bit more orange juice depending on how thick/thin you like your smoothies.

Serve immediately.

TIME	PREP TIME	SERVE
10m	10m	2

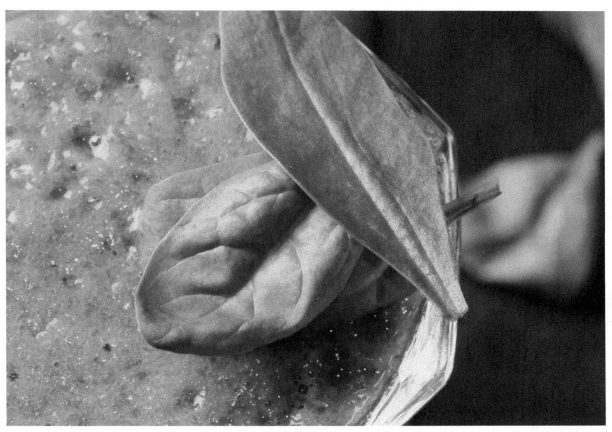

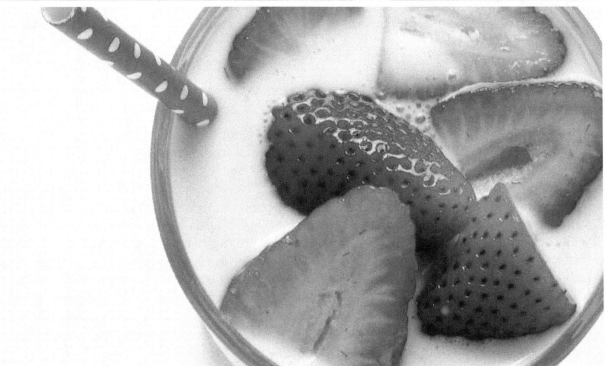

PEANUT BUTTER BANANA SMOOTHIE

Directions:

Place all ingredients into a high-speed blender.

Blend on high until smooth. Add more almond milk as needed.

Serve immediately.

Nutrition Facts

Serving Size: 1/2 Calories: 295 Sugar: 21 Fat: 10 Carbohydrates: 40 Fiber: 6 Protein: 12

Ingredients:

- 2 cups frozen sliced bananas
- 1/2 cup nonfat Greek yogurt
- 1/2 tablespoon ground flax seeds
- 1 cup unsweetened almond milk
- 1 teaspoon vanilla extract
- 2 tablespoons all-natural peanut

STRAWBERRY BANANA SPINACH SMOOTHIE

Ingredients:

- 2 cups frozen sliced bananas
- 2 cups frozen whole strawberries
- 4 cups fresh spinach
- 4 teaspoons chia seeds
- For serving (for 1 serving)
- 2 tablespoons vanilla protein powder (any kind)
- 1/2 cup unsweetened almond milk

Directions:

For the Bag First, line a baking sheet with parchment paper. Then, evenly spread out 2 cups of sliced bananas, 2 cups of whole strawberries. Place in the freezer for about 2 hours or until completely frozen. Next, take 4 quart-size freezer bags and write the date and Strawberry Banana Green Smoothie on the front. Add 1 cup of the frozen fruit, a handful of spinach, and a teaspoon of chia seeds to each bag. Before sealing, make sure you squeeze as much air out as possible to prevent freezer burn. Seal and place in the freezer for later use. For Blending (for 1 serving) Once you're ready to blend, empty contents of the spinach smoothie bag into a high-speed blender. Then, add about 1/2 cup of almond milk and 2 tablespoons of your favorite protein powder. Blend on High for about 1 minute or until everything is blended. Tips & Notes Nutrition information is for a single serving spinach smoothie. Storage: meal prep smoothie bags will stay for up to 3 months in the freezer. Option to double or triple this recipe. Nutrition Facts Serving Size: 1 smoothie Calories: 196 Sugar: 14 Fat: 4 Carbohydrates: 23 Fiber: 6 Protein: 16

TIME
10

PREP TIME
10

SERVE
2

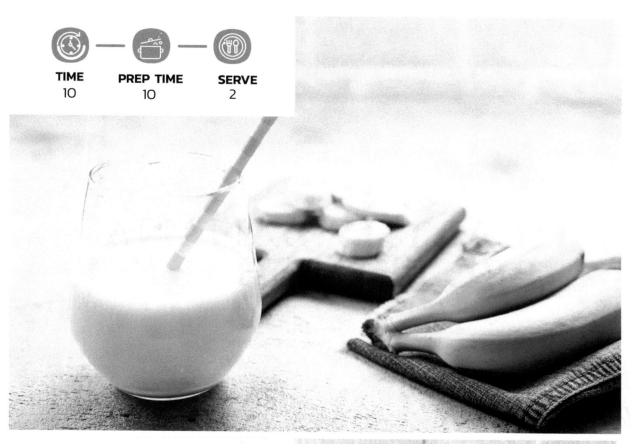

TIME
10m

PREP TIME
10m

SERVE
2

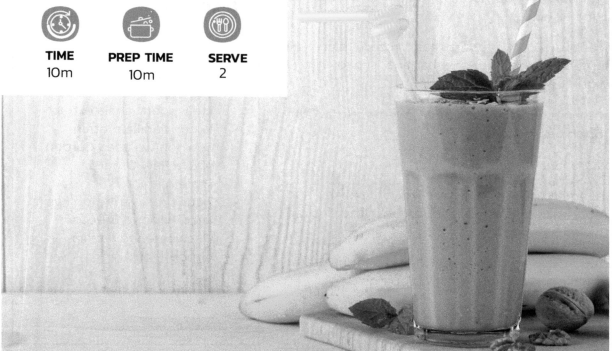

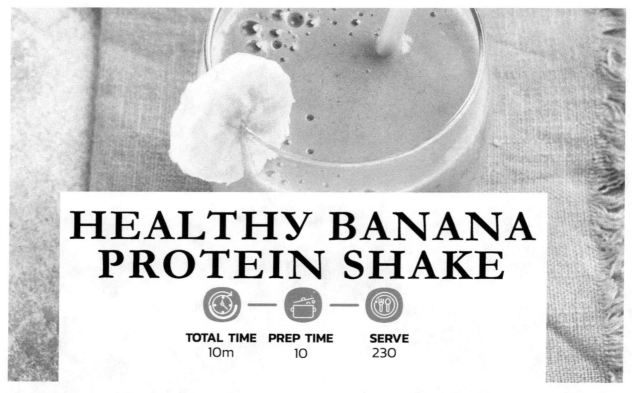

HEALTHY BANANA PROTEIN SHAKE

TOTAL TIME 10m

PREP TIME 10

SERVE 230

Directions:

First, freeze ¾ cup nonfat Greek Yogurt in an ice cube tray.

Once the Greek yogurt has frozen, place all ingredients for healthy banana shake into a high-speed blender.

Blend until smooth and serve with your favorite toppings.

Tips & Notes

Depending on how thick you like your shakes, add more milk by the tablespoon until the desired thickness is reached.

Nutrition does not include drizzled peanut butter or whipped coconut cream toppings.

nutrition: Serving Size: 1/4 recipe Calories: 163 Sugar: 10 Fat: 2 Carbohydrates: 19 Fiber: 3 Protein: 16

Ingredients:

- ¾ cup nonfat Greek yogurt, frozen into cubes
- 2 cups frozen sliced bananas
- 1 teaspoon vanilla extract
- ¼ cup vanilla protein powder (we used Garden of Life Raw Organic Protein)
- 2 cups milk, any kind (we used Almond Breeze Unsweetened Vanilla Almond Milk)

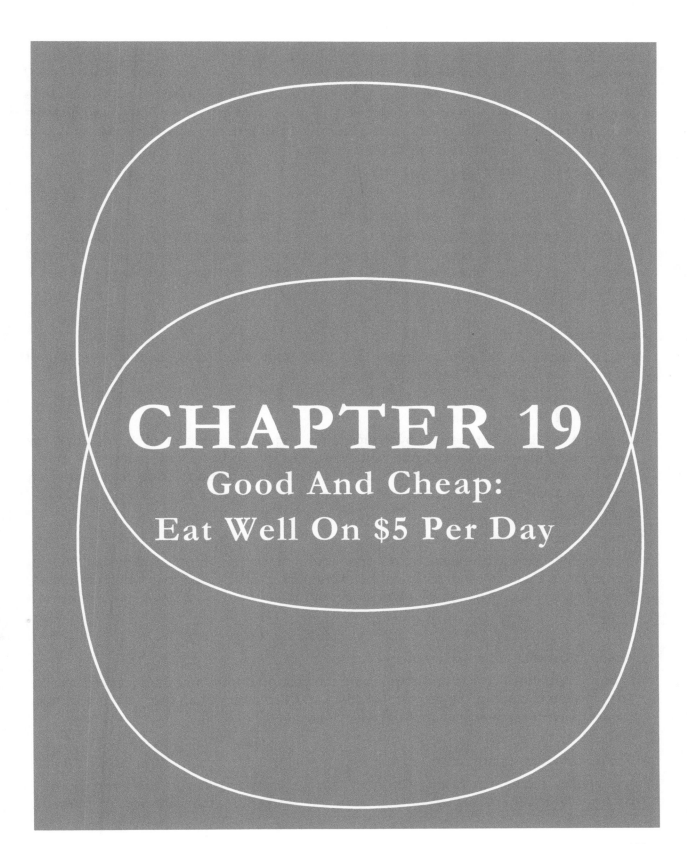

CHAPTER 19

Good And Cheap:
Eat Well On $5 Per Day

Have you ever heard anyone state that they don't eat a healthy diet because it's too expensive?

There is a lot of truth to that comment. Buying organic produce, grass-fed beef, free-range eggs, and various imported superfoods can be pricey. Add in all of the latest and greatest supplements, gluten-free baking, and a laundry list of must-have health food items, and your grocery bill is going to max out pretty quickly.

But, does healthy eating have to be like this?

How To Eat A Healthy Diet For Less Than $5 Per Day

I am a big-time eater. My job as a personal trainer is physical, and I burn many calories each Day. Unfortunately, this leads to a $600 per month grocery bill between my wife and myself (I take responsibility for the bulk of that obscene amount!) There has to be a diet that is healthy and much easier on the wallet. Let the search begin!

Requirements

Eating a "healthy" diet is quite subjective, so I created some requirements that must be met by my $5 per Day menu. They are as follows:

1. There must be enough calories.

Cutting the food bill would be easy by reducing the amount of food eaten each Day. But, there are so many reasons why it's important to eat enough food, so I don't want to skimp on calories. My goal was to create a daily diet that could provide up to 3,000 calories per Day and could easily offer the 2,000 calorie diet that most people need.

2. There must be enough protein.

High-protein foods can be expensive but are a crucial component of any healthy diet. Protein-dense foods are very filling, they help build and repair muscle, and they help promote fat-loss. My plan allows for well over 100 grams of protein per Day, which is plenty for most people.

3. Fruits and vegetables are mandatory.

This is non-negotiable. Fruits and veggies are the best nutrient-dense food source available. They are often lower in calories, high in fiber, and, like protein, can help us feel full much longer than processed carbs such as bread or pasta.

4. The diet must be balanced.

I have already alluded to this in my other rules, but I want to make sure this point is clear. A healthy diet offers a balance of protein, carbs, and fats. The idea that eating fat will make you fat is long-outdated (and never had much merit in the first place!), so a good diet must include healthy fat sources.

5. Meals must be easy to prepare.

This requirement has nothing to do with price. I don't have time to prepare meals for hours on end each Day, so I am looking for a relatively user-friendly menu. I want to do much of the prep work in bulk (before the week begins) so that the plan is easier to stick with when the busy work week hits.

My $5 Per Day Shopping List

I spent a lot of time calculating costs, nutritional values, calorie counts, etc., to develop a rough idea as to what foods I could include in my daily eating plan. Here are my final shopping list and the allotted quantities I portioned for one Day's worth of meals.

- Rolled oats (2 cups per Day, cooked)
- Almonds (15 per Day)
- Fruit – apples, pears, bananas (2 per Day)
- Whole grain brown rice (1 cup, cooked)
- Dried beans – chickpeas, kidney, black, navy, etc. (2 cups, cooked)
- Vegetables – Broccoli, cauliflower, sweet potatoes, onions, carrots, green peppers (4 servings)
- Tofu (100g)
- Quinoa (1 cup, cooked)
- All-natural peanut butter (2 tbsp)
- Tahini – used for homemade hummus (1/2 cup)
- Olive oil (2 tbsp)
- Whey protein (1 scoop)
- Why Did These Foods Make The Cut?

First off, these foods are all pretty inexpensive. A few items are a bit pricey (e.g., quinoa, almonds, peppers), but these can be cost-controlled by serving them in appropriate portions.

Proteins: Beans, quinoa, tofu, and why are all excellent protein sources and easily satisfied my requirement for at least 100g per Day.

Fats – Olive oil, almonds, peanut butter, tofu, and hummus offer an excellent range of fat sources that keep this daily diet balanced.

Calories: The fatty foods listed above are all calorie-dense and offer a good amount of energy for a relatively low cost. The same can be said for the whole grains chosen (oats, rice, and quinoa), which are also very versatile foods that can be used in many different dishes.

What Do I Do With These Ingredients?

This shopping list offers hundreds of potential meal ideas that can satisfy just about anyone's tastes. I added a range of spices to give flavor to some of the more bland foods (i.e., beans, rice, quinoa) and share some of those recipe ideas below.

I'm not going to prescribe a full meal plan here because eating on a budget like this should include some experimentation of your own. Take a little time to plan out your meals, test new spices, swap some ingredients, and you will find a list of meals that work for you.

Homemade Hummus
- 3 cups of chickpeas
- 3-5 tablespoons lemon juice (depending on taste)
- 2 tablespoons tahini
- 3 cloves garlic, crushed
- 1/2 teaspoon salt
- 2 tablespoons olive oil

Put the ingredients in a food processor or sturdy blender and blend until you reach your desired consistency. I used this hummus as a snack option along with raw carrots, broccoli, and cauliflower.

Cajun Beans and Rice Soup
Make your own Cajun spice using the following ingredients:
- 2 teaspoons salt
- 2 teaspoons garlic powder
- 2 1/2 teaspoons paprika
- 1 teaspoon ground black pepper
- 1 teaspoon onion powder
- 1 teaspoon cayenne pepper
- 1 1/4 teaspoons dried oregano
- 1 1/4 teaspoons dried thyme

The soup recipe is very easy once you have the right spice mix:
- 2 tablespoons olive oil
- 1 medium white onion, diced
- 1/2 medium green bell pepper, diced
- 2 cloves garlic, minced
- Cajun seasoning (as prepared above)

- 2 cups chicken broth
- 3 cups of water
- 3 cups kidney beans (cooked)
- 3 cups rice (cooked)

Cooking Instructions

1. Heat the olive oil in a large pot
2. Add the onion and garlic and let simmer for 2 minutes
3. Add the bell pepper and let simmer for another 2 minutes (the onion should not be semi-transparent)
4. Add all other ingredients, let it come to a boil, and then let simmer for 10 minutes

Chocolate Oatmeal

This is my go-to breakfast most mornings:

- 1 cup of rolled oats (cooked)
- 1 scoop of chocolate whey protein
- 15 almonds

So quick, easy, delicious, and filling!

And The Total Cost Is…?

The ingredients included in my shopping list brought my daily diet cost to $4.86. Keep in mind that this included very generous portions (and just over 3,000 calories per Day), but it did not include some staples that can be used long-term (i.e., spices, soup base mix).

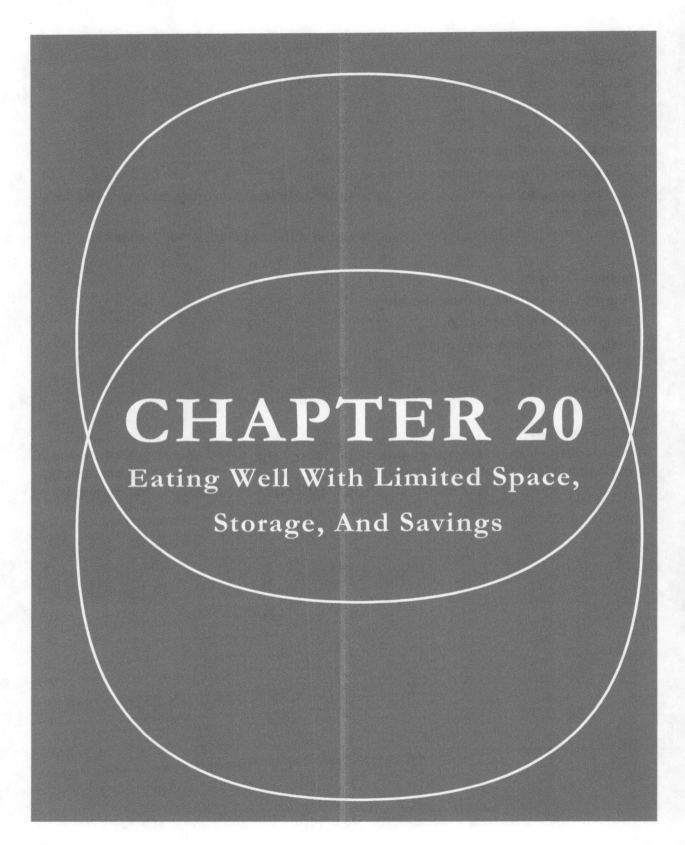

CHAPTER 20

Eating Well With Limited Space,
Storage, And Savings

While I've talked before about how we love purchasing food in bulk rather than in small, generally more expensive portions, this doesn't mean we have the ideal, organized pantry space with glass jars stacked on meticulously organized shelves. It doesn't mean we have a pantry at all.

Yes, I know I've talked about stocking my pantry on multiple occasions. However, in reality, our pantry consists of the kitchen's everyday cupboards, which already lack in size, and the counter below them that holds my dry containers. I also have a few limited shelving areas in the garage that provide food storage overflow. By limited, I mean one decent cupboard area where I store extra grains.

And that's it. In my opinion, not too shabby, but nothing spectacular either. It lacks in the storage department, especially when you consider the lack of any pantry or linen closet and that we spend the majority of our time cooking three or so times a day.

Making It Work

Here are a few of the things we've adjusted and adapted about our pantry-stocking style to make the limited space work for us.

- Make a pantry staples list.

Look through your cupboards and decide what the items you always need to have on hand are. Think about different flours, spices, grains, oils, and sauces that you use all the time. Those things you should always have on hand and will benefit from making room to store larger bulk-sized containers.

- Stock up only on the items you use frequently.

Similar to above, but it can include things like corn chips or your favorite dried fruits. For us, this means we purchase whole grains like quinoa in bulk and dried mangoes, but we stay away from perishable items that may not take as well to being stored in the fluctuating garage temperature or that we won't be eating in a relatively short period.

- Invest in storage containers that fit your space.

I love that Katie from Kitchen Stewardship uses whatever containers she comes across to hold her bulk goods. However, when working with limited space, a house with tiny or nonexistent closets, and an already overflowing storage area, we needed containers that were stacked and stored in that space we had. To hide the bulk goods we purchase, containers that slip into our cupboards maximize their potential, meaning we can stock up where it counts. (Example: a 10-pound bag of organic quinoa costs the same as the 2-pound.)

These are just methods that help us minimize clutter in our 1,100-square-foot house. There was a lot of giving and take when we moved to this house, as our last house had a fantastic pantry closet that we used for all of our kitchen appliances, as well as food storage.

Finding what worked in this space took a year or two of testing with plenty of successes and failures. For you, the answer may be different. How do you determine where to stock up and save and be less frugal and more organizationally-minded?

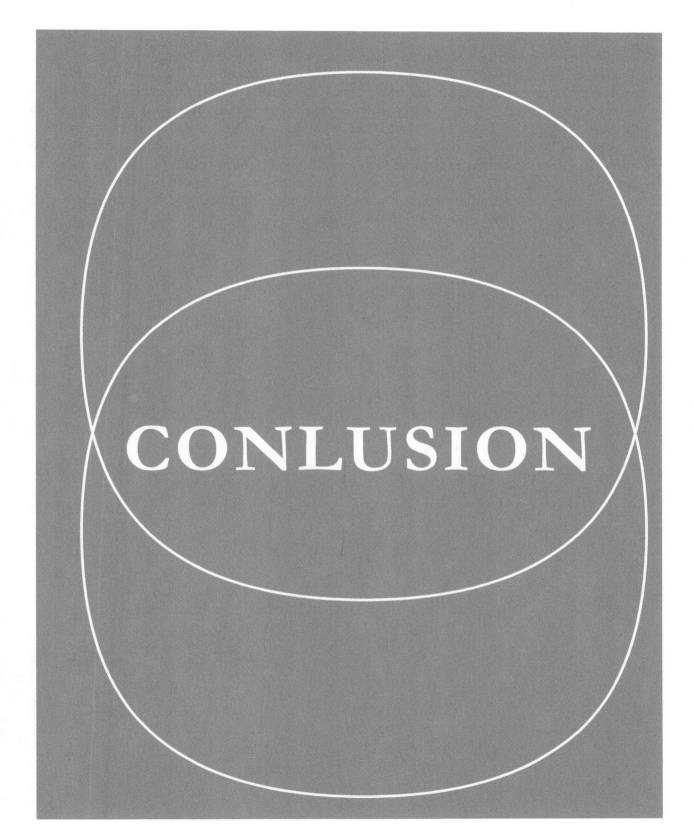

CONLUSION

Tiny fridge, a tiny budget, big appetite—a college student's guide to eating well. Early classes, final exams, and the occasional party—college students have enough on their plate without worrying about putting food on it. The Budget-Friendly College Cookbook is your go-to guide for nutritionally navigating your college years on your own with tasty meals like Chicken French Bread Pizza and Pesto Pasta in a Mug that require minimal appliances and ingredients. Learn to cook on a very small budget, put your limited space to good use, and even avoid that notorious Freshman 15. Many of these college cookbook recipes take less than five minutes to prepare, from breakfast to desserts, make use of ingredients that don't require refrigeration, and are geared toward small portions. Walk away from college with a lifetime degree in a low-cost nutritional lifestyle.

CPSIA information can be obtained
at www.ICGtesting.com
Printed in the USA
BVHW052014300321
603712BV00004B/248

9 781802 346947